I'M SORRY, IT'S CANCER:

A HANDBOOK OF HELP AND HOPE FOR SURVIVORS AND CAREGIVERS

I'M SORRY, IT'S CANCER:

A HANDBOOK OF HELP AND HOPE FOR SURVIVORS AND CAREGIVERS

CHRIS FREY, MSW

Foreword by
DR. LANNIS HALL, MD, MPH

ISBN 978-1-257-00692-2

What People Are Saying About Chris Frey's...

I'M SORRY, IT'S CANCER:
A Handbook of Help and Hope for Survivors and Caregivers

"This is a comprehensive battle plan to combat cancer. I'm impressed with the thoughtful approach to all the aspects of the cancer journey. All too often patients are overwhelmed or have trouble finding help. This is a how-to guide for them...Perhaps most enlightening was the recovery section...Sometimes the aftermath is harder than battling the actual disease."

Dave, cancer survivor

"Chris Frey has written from his heart and from his experience as a person diagnosed with cancer. He shares his journey of navigating the health care system, getting social support and gaining life perspective. Frey, a social worker and relationship specialist, demonstrates gratitude for the care he received by sharing insights from his cancer journey with readers. If you are looking for an autobiographical self-help cancer handbook written in conversational style, this is the book for you."

Mercedes Bern-Klug, PhD, MSW, Assistant Professor: University of Iowa School of Social Work, Aging Studies Program

"I'M SORRY, IT'S CANCER is truly a handbook that can be referred to at each step of the cancer journey – diagnosis, during treatment and post-treatment. I felt the sections on building a care team were particularly helpful. Even if you don't have a built-in care team with family members close by, you can build a team of physicians, nurses, social workers, co-workers and friends, and access local cancer organizations to work with you through your journey. Mr. Frey's book is a great companion for those on the cancer journey. His book

provides helpful advice, real life suggestions and caveats for anyone with a cancer diagnosis. His real life experience as both a social worker and a cancer patient puts him in a unique position to offer significant help."

Laura Rossmann, Executive Director, the Wellness Community of Greater St. Louis

"I'M SORRY, IT'S CANCER is an inspirational book that asks the right questions to help the survivor and caregiver know if they are on the right track to comprehensive care-- both physically and emotionally. Chris Frey covers many areas in ways not covered in other cancer books-- support, advocacy, assertiveness, joy, grief, giving back, the male perspective. I wish this book had been around when my mother was diagnosed."

Connie, caregiver and Licensed Clinical Social Worker

"Chris' words validate the thoughts people have as being "normal" and gives positive insights on what actions people can take to assume control of what often seems like an uncontrollable situation. Chris shares his own experiences, thoughts and ideas on how to make the best of the cancer journey. He does this with humor and respect. I recommend this easy to read book to all new cancer patients as a road guide through the cancer journey."

Sharon Lee, RN, BSN, Manager, Siteman Cancer Center at Barnes-Jewish St. Peters Hospital

"This book puts the struggle against cancer within a larger framework, one in which inspiration and hope are not based on denial but on emotional honesty and down-to-earth advice."

Serge Prengel, author of Resolutions That Work

"Chris Frey offers a treasure of wisdom, insight, and meaning in this personal account of his struggle through cancer. Chris brings together profound self-reflection, a warm and engaging style of writing and the best suggestions I've seen for psychological and spiritual resources for facing cancer. Chris is a writer who can fruitfully bring together an impeccable career as a psychotherapist with a personal journey

rich with compassion and help to others. I highly recommend this wonderful book."

Terry D. Cooper, EdD, PhD, Professor of Psychology and author of Making Judgments without Being Judgmental, Paul Tillich and Psychology, and Reinhold Niebuhr and Psychololgy

"Chris Frey provides concrete yet empathetic suggestions to help survivors navigate the emotionally charged road to survival and recovery."

Mark Tobin, LPC, CCMHC

To DiAnne, Carly, Aimee, and Nathan:
You give me purpose and joy.

To Joyce: you taught me what being a survivor means.
You showed me the way.

To the survivors, family members, friends, professionals,
and volunteers who walked with me on this part of my
journey. You remind me that each day is precious.

ACKNOWLEGEMENTS

Utmost gratitude to Dr. Lannis Hall for writing the Foreword and for her incredible dedication to the health and well-being of cancer survivors and their families.

Many thanks to my wife, DiAnne, Chris Scribner, PhD, Connie Fisher, LCSW and Mary Schanuel of the Synergy Group for your assistance in editing and improving the manuscript. You helped me change the book I imagined into the book that needed to be written.

This book was made possible, in part, through a grant from the Armour Foundation. A special thanks to Terry, Jim, Dude and Shirley.

To all of the staff at The Siteman Cancer Center-St. Peters, the Center for Advanced Medicine and Barnes Hospital, my eternal gratitude.

Thanks to my friends on the Patient and Family Advisory Council, who encourage and teach me day after day. It's wonderful to sit with folks who truly celebrate the value of each life.

CONTENTS

FOREWORD

The diagnosis of cancer can be the most difficult challenge in one's life. Accepting that a once normal cell has turned malignant and now threatens your survival is an incredibly difficult concept to absorb. Approximately 1.5 million Americans face this tragic situation each year but through steady improvements in treatment approximately 70 percent of these men and women will successfully overcome their disease. This improvement in survival has increased from 50 percent of men and women at five years in the 1970's and is directly attributable to early detection and improved therapies.

Chris Frey has beautifully detailed the importance of building your team, the necessity of emotional and physical support, and seeking state of the art care to successfully conquer this disease. I am humbled daily by the opportunity to play such an important role in my patients' lives. We meet in a valley and I am called upon to provide treatment expertise, supportive resources and encouragement critical to a successful outcome. Throughout the book, Chris highlights the importance of being an active participant in one's healthcare and recognizing that maintaining a healthy lifestyle after treatment is crucial to feeling well and preventing recurrence.

Chris has done what all of us should aspire for in life. He has taken a personal tragedy, conquered it, and given us his road map to recovery. Thank you, Chris, for giving profoundly of yourself and improving the lives of many future cancer patients.

Lannis Hall, MD, MPH
Director of Radiation Oncology
Barnes-Jewish St. Peters Hospital

Assistant Professor of Medicine
Clinical Radiation Oncology
Washington University School of Medicine

THAT DAY

"We knew from the moment of diagnosis that coping with cancer would require the strength and support of many people. We began reaching out immediately."

Survivor and Caregiver

"I'm sorry, it's cancer."

I don't remember the day of the week, or what I was wearing, or the weather. But, I remember those four words as vividly as if the doctor had just spoken them. I've heard words like "remission," and "all clear" since that day. Wonderful words, powerful words. Yet for now and ever, in that moment, I became a cancer survivor.

You Are Not Alone

You or a loved one may have just heard those four words. As you read, you may be sitting in the waiting room of a doctor's office, clinic or hospital. Perhaps you are awaiting a complete diagnosis, developing a treatment plan, already engaged in medical intervention, or even entering into a post-treatment phase of your recovery. Whatever your situation, I want you to know that *you are not alone*.

This handbook is provided as one resource to help survivors and families find, and fully utilize, the people and support services that will empower you for the journey through cancer. I offer my experience as a fellow survivor and family member, blended with 30 years as a social worker and psychotherapist, in this brief and practical guide for maximizing the quality of the physical, emotional and spiritual care necessary to restore your family to health. At every turn, through the most difficult days of recovery, I found professionals, family, old friends, new friends and spiritual comfort that sustained me. I hope the words that follow will help you do the same.

Throughout these pages I will offer questions and practical suggestions for your consideration. Many of these will be highlighted in color. Pause...Take a little time to consider each. You may choose to write in a journal and reflect on my ideas in your own words. When able, discuss your thoughts and feelings with people you trust. The answers you find will greatly assist you in locating the resources that provide the highest measure of independence and control as you travel this path.

The book is divided into four sections: *The Journey Begins; Building a Care Team; Treatment and Recovery;* and *Aftercare.* Each contains recommendations on a wide range of topics pertinent to your situation. I encourage you to enter into this information at whatever point best meets your needs. This guide is for you.

Most often, I will speak directly to the person facing cancer. I will use the word "survivor" when I refer to anyone who has been diagnosed, or is in any stage of the recovery process. From the first day the words "it's cancer" are spoken, each of us becomes a survivor of this disease. This is a term of dignity and strength.

If you are a family member, professional, or other advocate, the ideas I discuss are designed to also assist you in understanding the experience and needs of those you care for. I hope my words will help take you further inside the world of the survivors in your life.

THE JOURNEY BEGINS

"Look out for yourself, because nobody else does is not a correct characterization of family, friends and medical staff in the broad scope of cancer care. In addition to the survivors, themselves, people will help however they can."

Survivor

Coping with Diagnosis

I was a pretty healthy guy at the tender age of fifty-two. Then one fine summer morning I woke up, stretched, rubbed my neck and felt a small lump on the right side, just under my chin. I did the right thing. I called my primary care physician, a great guy I've known for years. I scheduled an appointment. Other than the lump, the only other symptom I was aware of was a bit of extra fatigue, which I had written off as "Most busy folks my age have some fatigue." The doctor prescribed an antibiotic and gave me a referral to an Ear, Nose and Throat specialist, in the event I was dealing with something more serious than an infection.

Three doctors, less than a month's time, a neck biopsy and a throat scope later, I was sitting in that ENT's consultation room with my wife DiAnne. After the various poking and prodding I'd recently experienced, we both knew what we might hear that day. For several weeks my internal conversations had moved from "Don't jump to conclusions" to "What if...?" I had imagined other relatively simple outcomes. Perhaps a little benign cyst. Maybe I was going to need additional medication, or outpatient surgery. My wishful thinking included "maybe it will just go away."

"I'm sorry, it's cancer."

The next thing I recall, through a fog of shock and fear of hearing those four words, is turning and looking into DiAnne's eyes. Not at all what we had hoped to hear. I think DiAnne said "I'm so sorry honey," but I'm not sure.

I do remember the doctor telling me I was not in any of the high-risk groups for this type of cancer. It didn't matter. Here we were. Squamous cell, a spot in my throat and lymph nodes in the right side of my neck. Stage 4: a piece of information I would manage not to register until I read it in a letter several days later. A CAT scan and PET scan would soon prove this to be only a partial diagnosis. Further testing found cancerous nodes on the left side of my neck.

Now, it seems as if an instant passed from doctor's diagnosis and initial recommendations to DiAnne and me standing in the clinic parking lot.

Tears. Confusion. Questions. Lots of questions. Although DiAnne and I had both worked in the field of healthcare and previously had supported family members on the journey through cancer, we had absolutely no knowledge of my specific type of cancer. We were truly out of our element.

One message from the doctor had been absolutely clear, though. While my situation was not urgent, I was dealing with an advanced, aggressive cancer and we needed to get moving.

And so where do we go from here? More tests. Surgery, perhaps by a surgeon she had recommended. Radiation on the right side of my neck. But what surgery? Should it be the surgeon recommended by the ENT, who we barely knew? Radiation? What type? Where? When? Would there be other treatment? How would we tell the kids? What about insurance? What about my business? Would I be able to speak after throat surgery? Would I recover? As you may know, for a time, the questions come much quicker than the answers.

To some small degree I calmed myself in that parking lot on that day based on four decisions made with my number one advocate and caregiver, DiAnne. First, she would immediately call close friends Jim and Nanci, who we knew had considerable knowledge about the best physicians and medical treatment in our community. Second, we would make the most of the brief time available to check out the full range of care options open to me. Third, I would call my business partner Mark who is, among other wonderful things, a calm and wise man. Fourth, we would tell our children Carly, Aimee and Nathan about my diagnosis only after outlining an initial plan of action.

Amidst the flood of questions and emotions, this plan was the first step in moving from *Why Me?* to *What Next?* Please know that you and your loved ones may cover this territory many times in the days ahead. That's OK.

You are not alone.

Your Journey

Each of us has our own unique story of how this trip began, a moment that may be frozen in time. The emotions you and your family are feeling and the decisions you are facing may be beyond any you have previously confronted in your life.

Today, what matters most to me is that my story is a shared story. I was not alone.

DiAnne was the first and most magnificent of literally dozens of advocates and caregivers who have encouraged, nurtured and challenged me in every phase of my recovery. I emphatically suggest that, like me, choosing the people who will assist you in creating the plan that fortifies your fighting spirit is an essential first step toward health.

We know that the rates of surviving cancer continue to increase as the field advances. We also know that a strong support system increases our follow through with treatment, which ensures that each of us has the best possible chance of recovery.

Cancer calls upon each of us to assemble a team that not only provides the best medical care we can generate but also the personal support that helps us maintain our motivation and internal strength through the days to come. The emotions and complex series of decisions that come with a diagnosis of cancer can seem overwhelming, for survivors and caregivers alike. The time we have to process these emotions and make these essential decisions is limited. And so the support network we create becomes vital through each stage of this challenge. The team may include medical professionals, family, old friends, new friends, volunteers, community agencies and for many of us, faith in a universal power.

> What are the most immediate decisions that face you in this moment?
>
> In consultation with medical experts, what is a realistic timeline for making decisions about your medical treatment plan, insurance, other financial issues and the needs of your family?
>
> What are your family's emotional and spiritual concerns?
>
> What other issues are unique to your situation?

We begin to find answers to these questions by opening ourselves to all available resources.

Understanding Your Needs at Diagnosis: Physical and More

"What would you recommend to a client of yours in this situation, Chris?"

"I'd say the doctor's recommendation seems like a good idea."

"How about we give that a try, then."

This is my recollection of the input of a good friend, when I resisted one of my physician's recommendations. I agreed to try the doctor's idea. It turned out to be a good one.

Opening Our Hearts

Building a complete care system calls us to creativity, research and an open heart. As, you may already know, cancer is distinctive in the wide range of people it affects. Children, adolescents and adults of every age, from all walks of life, cope with this illness. Further, the word itself, cancer, is an umbrella term that denotes a vast array of types and subtypes, each of which is impacted by the ever-evolving nature of diagnosis and treatment. In the past week alone I learned of new discoveries in research on breast cancer and a specific form of brain cancer. In its breadth and complexity, cancer demands interpersonal resources that will take us through each stage of treatment, and beyond.

You may be a person who easily reaches out to others for help. You may be a very independent soul, even someone who resists the help of others.

Cancer changes the rules. The multi-level support system you build will be essential for the fight ahead.

Information: Research and Preparing for Treatment

The myriad categories of information that affected the course of my recovery included diagnosis, medical treatment, medications, managing the side effects of treatment, nutrition, exercise, medical supplies, insurance, business and financial concerns, legal information, social services, stress management, emotional coping skills, spiritual support, child and family stress.

The people resources that I relied on to help gather and interpret the volume of information vital to my recovery included physicians, physicians assistants, nurses, nursing assistants, social workers, billing staff, radiation technologists, physicists, a nutritionist, a speech pathologist, clergy, psychotherapists, a dentist, a dental hygienist, community volunteers, local cancer agency staff, home health care, medical supply staff, other survivors, my wife, my children, my siblings, my parents, my sister-in-law, other extended family members, numerous friends, the Internet and the Siteman-St. Peters Cancer Center Patient and Family Advisory Council, of which I am a member.

For example, I was encouraged to see my dentist before initiating treatment. The products his staff gave me to use during radiation were enormously helpful in protecting my teeth and mouth, a part of the plan I would not have known to include without research by my wife and the recommendations of a knowledgeable person in our community. This was not my most pressing decision but one that has paid dividends in the aftercare stage of my recovery.

Looking back, I realize that even with all these talented experts in my corner, I missed significant information and at times suffered undue pain. The technical nature and sheer amount of data presented to us cannot be digested without assistance. Imagine, then, the potential cost if we isolate and disconnect?

As I hear the stories of other survivors, I am reminded that there are multiple styles for gathering vital information. One size does not fit all. Some folks want every morsel of potentially useful data from every external source available. Some of us do varying degrees of our own research. Along this continuum are those who let it be known that we want the medical experts to provide only the basic information necessary to determine a plan of treatment.

> As you read this book, begin to develop a list of informational needs unique to your situation. What are the questions that are most pressing for you? Write them down. Bring them to your appointments. Make sure each is answered in a way that makes sense to you and your advocates.

More questions will occur to you over time. Identify the resources around you: books, treatment staff, the Internet, other survivors, which can assist you as treatment evolves.

Advocates also differ in the need for information. My wife did a great deal of her own research. Other caregivers report a less active process. What are the informational needs of your primary caregivers? Write them down. Bring them to appointments.

Whatever the stage on your road through recovery, take a moment to consider the people and places (library, Internet, cancer care agencies, other community services) that can be sources of additional, valuable information.

Ask yourself who you already know that may have expert, or at least wise, counsel on the resources you will need over time. Who is already on your team? Who has come into your world for the specific purpose of advancing your path through cancer?

Physical Support: More than Medicine

Physical support comes in many forms: the actual medical care we receive, assistance with our activities of daily living, transportation, financial assistance and so much more. Physical support also includes the people who reach out to our families when they need respite, caring for us as our loved ones take time for themselves. Trust and confidence in those who provide this care is a powerful component in maintaining our dignity and optimism.

Now I am not an unusually modest or self-conscious guy, but the number of strangers or near strangers who viewed and tested various parts of my body during diagnosis, treatment and beyond must rival what occurs for a newborn, a stage of life I don't remember very well. My reliance on others to assist me in daily life functions that I have taken for granted as easy tasks for a healthy person was both humbling and greatly appreciated.

A strong personal support system and the inner circle of your medical team become tremendous assets in offsetting what at times seems like enormous invasions of your private space and independence.

Some of us will need to draw on friends and nonmedical advocates outside of our immediate family for practical assistance. Your family resources may be limited or the demands of your situation may simply become more than family can manage. Immediately after returning home from surgery, I required around-the-clock care. I needed assistance to walk, administer medication, take in nutrition and shower. Over time, DiAnne and I turned to extended family and old friends for transportation, meals, night watch, lawn care, mail delivery and more.

> What are your physical care needs at this time?
>
> What needs do you anticipate as you look forward?
>
> Who is available?
>
> Who is available beyond immediate family that can assist you and give respite to your primary caregivers?

During diagnosis it is impossible to know every need you will have, or every resource you will require for the journey. As you continue to identify the physical assistance you need, open your heart and ask for additional help. You may be amazed at the practical support available to you.

Emotional Support: Coping with Diagnosis and Sustaining Motivation

Cancer put me in touch with every feeling I am aware of. In my travels, other survivors and family members have shared their stories of anger, fear, guilt, sadness and confusion. Why me? Why didn't I take better care of myself? How will my appearance change? What is my prognosis? Who will take care of me? Who will take care of my family? The emotions that follow our questions and concerns during diagnosis and treatment can be rapid and relentless.

It can be particularly difficult to make the series of complex decisions required by a cancer diagnosis when your loved ones and you are still reeling from the emotions that often accompany this devastating news. Your feelings can be impacted by the type of cancer you are experiencing, the stage and prognosis of your illness, the timeline you face to make decisions about medical care, the responses of caregivers, and many other factors.

These feelings, at varying levels of intensity, can significantly color our verbal and nonverbal interactions with medical staff, other caregivers, even the person who tells us the doctor is running late. They impact motivation, energy and hope.

Feelings can turn to depression and anxiety. Feelings can also fuel motivation and tenacity. Finding ways to identify and express the full range of emotion is essential to maximizing our internal resources, increasing our responsiveness to the care of others, and enhancing the general health of survivors and caregivers. Avoiding or denigrating our feelings can significantly interfere with the ability to connect and communicate with loved ones and professionals, especially when we are in physical distress, or when we have received painful news about our cancer.

A few straightforward tools can help:

Become aware of basic feelings: anger, sadness, fear, hurt, happiness, guilt, embarrassment. If you are unaware of what you are feeling, ask for a trusted advocate to help you identify the current emotion.

Become aware of changes in your behavior and mood, such as increased irritability, self-criticism, low energy not caused by medical treatment, difficulty eating or sleeping. These and other changes often are symptoms of emotional challenges.

Share feelings as they occur, in smaller doses, rather than saving your pain until it is overwhelming. Unexpressed annoyance and frustration can build to deep levels of anger, anxiety and depression which interfere with motivation and energy.

Consult with your treatment team about emotional changes and their effects on your progress.

Tell yourself that each feeling has been experienced by numerous other survivors and caregivers.

Become aware of how your feelings affect your attitude, positively and negatively, about treatment and recovery.

Share your fears and frustrations with other survivors and caregivers, as many times as necessary.

Endeavor to remember who is on your side. If you express anger in a way that is detrimental to a caregiver, or to yourself, take responsibility and move on.

Find one or more people who will listen to your optimism and hope and faith, and celebrate your victories.

Identify and utilize those who can handle talking about the tough stuff.

There is no doubt that some of us are blessed with spouses, partners, parents and adult children who provide powerful emotional comfort. I count myself especially fortunate to include my wife, my sister and my sister-in-law on the list of people who are gifted at the art of care giving. However, DiAnne and I live in a city where we are many miles away from all biological family. Family came when they could, but there were many months when cultivating a circle of nonfamily caregivers was absolutely essential to our journey through cancer.

Creating a complete system of emotional allies provides us and our loved ones with necessary breathing space, along with multiple outlets for stress and worry. In the aftermath of diagnosis, I consulted numerous family, friends, and colleagues on issues ranging from medical care to temporarily closing my business to strategies for helping our children cope.

Early in treatment, it was Fran, Marilyn, Lisa and my parents who sat and listened to me so DiAnne could go to work or get a few hours of sleep. Later Jim drove 100 miles every Tuesday to transport me to my clinic. He helped me create a guided imagery to comfort my anxiety during radiation. Doug drove me downtown for follow-up and kept me company on one very long day in my surgeon's waiting room. As soon as I was able, Ralph walked with me every Sunday and listened to my laundry list of complaints. Mark, my business partner of twenty years, brought his calmness and wise consult to my entire family from that first day, up to the present. Connie listened, sat with me as I cried, and kept watch as I slept.

The special people in our lives not only provide us with practical assistance, they attend to our hearts and spirits. This is absolutely necessary as we adjust to the realities of diagnosis and fight to heal. You may already know who these people are. It is simply a matter of opening the door.

Some of you face serious limitations within your caregiver system. Perhaps your primary support people are aging or experiencing their own health concerns. You may live in somewhat isolated circumstances, geographically removed from caregivers. Key relationships in your life may be conflictual or distant. Your family members may not have the physical or emotional capacity to provide a high level of care. Or you may simply be an introverted person who has functioned independently without a significant need for close interpersonal connection.

And so you may be wondering, "How will I find these allies?"

Read on.

One of my favorite sayings to other survivors and cancer treatment professionals is, "Many of my friends are therapists and I recommend everybody get themselves a couple. They often know just what to do and say when I am scared, angry, sad, confused and happy." In short, the empathy, compassion and clarity offered by those we turn to for counsel is an indispensable part of a powerful cancer recovery strategy.

Therapists come in many forms. Some are trained professionals. They may even specialize in work with cancer survivors and families. Individual, group and family counseling all have a useful place in many of our treatment plans. Public and private insurance often pays for at least a portion of these services. Many communities offer public and church funded agencies, and even some private pay therapists, that operate on a sliding fee scale; the cost of services is adjusted based on income.

Many cancer treatment centers provide a combination of lay and professional services for coping with the stress of diagnosis, treatment and beyond, often at minimal or no cost. These services might include group support for survivors by type of cancer, groups on healing meditation and guided imagery, medication for depression and anxiety, seminars on coping with side effects, and workshops on everything from nutrition and exercise to body image and sexuality. I recently learned of a wonderful colleague who is specializing in play therapy with children who are cancer survivors, helping them cope with the emotional impact of their illness.

Another resource is clergy, some of whom have special training in counseling and a capacity for great compassion. For many of us, a clergy person may be the first place we would comfortably turn in this time of emotional and spiritual hardship.

Other folks are simply what I call 'natural healers.' These are the friends, family and fellow life travelers who are innately rich in providing comfort. They listen well and are especially adept in times of crisis. Often they are other survivors and advocates who understand our struggles on a deep personal level.

Some of you already have an abundance of these people in your life. For you, it is a matter of inviting those who are interested to accompany you on the path. You may need to make the phone calls, send the emails and ask for help. Or you may only need to say "Yes;" upon hearing on your situation, people will find you.

Once again, some of you face special challenges in creating the circle of care that will sustain you through these difficult times. In the next chapter I will offer more detailed suggestions on identifying and connecting with key resource people.

Here are a few initial thoughts:

> It's OK to ask for help. If you are a very independent or introverted person this will be what some of my friends call "a stretch," pushing yourself beyond your comfort zone.

> It's OK to reach beyond family. You may not have an extensive or stable family to draw on for certain aspects of your care. Cancer care is a community effort and resources are expanding to people from all walks of life.

> Let yourself know that there are people who want to help. It is your role to identify them and ask for what you need. They may be casual acquaintances, folks from the workplace, old friends and new, community caregivers and volunteers.

These allies listen to our complaints, provide messages of hope, offer solace, function as sounding boards, give practical input when asked and provide relief for our primary caregivers. Perhaps best of all, these people hold us in their hearts and their arms as we heal and struggle.

Social Support

Through the course of treatment, I did not always want to talk about cancer. Sometimes we, as survivors and caregivers, want or need to take a walk, talk about our kids' achievements, hear about our friends' daily lives, laugh a bit. Almost any meaningful conversation can include health issues, but cancer does not have to dominate every moment or every relationship.

My wonderful sister-in-law Joyce loved to ride horses, talk about horses and care for horses. And she did all of that, throughout her journey through cancer. One of my immensely joyful memories is watching my wife and my sisters-in-law, Joyce and Marilyn (three elegant women), dress up in mud clothes and trek down to the barn to feed the horses.

I also remember a survivor who, when able, continued to travel with his spouse. I know a woman who is the ultimate hockey mom and a caregiver who is active in dog rescue. When I was able, I went out with friends for smoothies, attended school functions and went to the movies. Now I go to community events, meeting survivors and caregivers at every stage in the journey, visiting, sharing stories, giving hugs, crying, laughing.

And I often recall a special day, soon after returning home from surgery, when the in-home social worker came to visit. These were some of the most painful days of my treatment. I was exhausted and only partially coherent. Early in the meeting, my wife cleverly shared that I was a social worker and writer. The visiting social worker asked me about my work and my books. She was genuinely interested in our common experiences. For just a little while, I was reminded that I was more than a patient, more than my pain. That was our only contact. I will never forget that woman.

Social support, then, blends with emotional support to ease the struggles of cancer and enrich our world beyond illness. As you move through recovery, consider the people, places and activities that bring you comfort, pleasure, distraction and a sense of accomplishment.

> Who and what reinforces your positive self-worth?
>
> Who and what reminds you that you are a survivor or caregiver, and much more?
>
> Who takes you seriously?
>
> Who helps you laugh?

From social support comes hope, encouragement, and in the best of times, a respite from the often all-encompassing challenge that cancer can become.

Spiritual Support: Through Diagnosis and Beyond

I believe that all assistance we receive in difficult times has a spiritual component. Acts of caring remind us that we are connected to some greater good and that at its core, life is about relationships. The nature and scope of these relationships may vary significantly among us, impacted by family, friends, race, ethnicity, spiritual or religious beliefs and more. What does not vary is our basic human desire for connection.

I have found many of my fellow cancer survivors to be individuals of deep conviction and faith. How else do we trust in the steadiness of a surgeon's hands and heart, after only moments of consultation? How else do we enter, day after day, into the trials of ongoing treatment with enough hope to balance our fear and frustration? How else do we persevere in the face of inconclusive or negative test results?

Spiritual support might come from your religious faith. You may tap into an even deeper reliance on long-held beliefs, or return to an earlier faith. I have seen religious communities draw together to provide all measure of support to people in need, from prayer to the very practical assistance of meals, transportation, fund raising and child care. For many families, this community of faith is absolutely essential on the path through cancer.

Some of us find hope and healing in our relationship with, as named in the "12 Step" self-help program, a power greater than ourselves. This powerful sense of a healing presence in our lives may or may not be attached to any specific faith or doctrine.

During diagnosis and therapy, my family and I received Protestant prayers of many denominations, Catholic prayers and Jewish prayers. I was told by my sister that a Native American water pourer led a Native sweat lodge and prayer circle in my honor. The pastor of my church reached out repeatedly to me and to my family. A wonderful friend and pastor prayed and brought the positive energy of Reiki to my recovery. One wonderful old friend told me, "I don't pray, but I'm praying for you." I welcomed them all. Each reminded me that there are mysteries and miracles in illness and health and healing that no one, not even the most skilled physician or learned clergy, can fully explain.

Cancer most assuredly tests our hope and faith. Mine has certainly not been constant or unbending, especially when first diagnosed and during the most rigorous times of each form of treatment. Still, the courage, willpower and tenacity that I have witnessed among fellow survivors and family members is beyond my full comprehension and, for me, only seems possible through the combined energy of gutsy individuals, loving communities and inspiration drawn from spirit.

Many of you are clear about the ways you will rely on your faith to fortify you as you enter active treatment. For those who are open to investigating the value of spirit in your treatment and recovery, these questions may help:

What belief system do you carry with regard to a spiritual life that will provide strength during difficult times and celebration in times of victory?

Does the challenge of cancer present you with an opportunity to renew, deepen, or for the first time explore spiritual and religious beliefs?

Do your values bring you hope, peace and encouragement?

How might your current beliefs serve you in expanding your network of support?

Do your current views interfere with your willingness or ability to reach out to others, or prevent potential advocates from extending themselves to you? If so, who would be available to assist you if you expand your vision of spirit?

Have you closed your circle to only those who share your way of life, or have you opened your heart to the enrichment that comes from allowing new resources into your life?

What additional help is available to you as you enlarge your view of physical, emotional and spiritual support?

As survivors, our interpersonal world is a beautiful mixture of family backgrounds, races, genders and belief systems. Now is not the time for debate. Now is the time for acceptance and open hearts.

What and who do you believe in? Yourself? Family? Friends? Medicine? A higher being? Miracles? I encourage you to consider which of these have a place in your recovery.

This brings us to putting our faith in the highest quality of medical care we can find.

BUILDING YOUR CARE TEAM

"As I began the cancer journey, I remembered a saying my high school basketball coach would use. The team would huddle up close in a circle with one hand raised, our heads touching together. In unison we would say, "Together We Attack!" I really took him to heart after my diagnosis and thrived on the team approach with my support members-my spouse, family, friends, co-workers, doctors, nurses and other caregivers- to push hard every day. I expected the collective strength of the team to achieve results much higher than going on this journey alone."

Survivor

Medical Care:
It Can Be Who You Know

"If this were someone you loved, what would you do?"

This is a question my wife asked one of the physicians we consulted. The doctor's answer was compassionate and specific. We chose this person to become a part of my treatment.

Finding the Best Care Available

I was told in the early stages of diagnosis that I would need surgery and radiation on the right side of my neck. Through further testing, I soon learned that radiation on both sides, plus chemotherapy, were recommended. As news of the seriousness of my condition accelerated, my anxiety and sense of urgency kept pace. It was essential to find the best care within the limited time available.

We immediately began the search for the best medical team available. The agreed upon call from DiAnne to our friends yielded the name of a local pioneer in oral cancer surgery. These wonderful people assisted us in making contact. After a bit of effort navigating the channels of a large city teaching hospital, we found ourselves meeting with Dr. Bruce Haughey, MBChB, MS, FACS, FRACS, a man I now call, "my surgeon." Within one consultation, I made a commitment to allow this physician to perform laser surgery on my throat and a bi-lateral neck dissection for cancerous lymph nodes. I had agreed in very short order to put my life in the hands of a doctor with whom I had never had a cup of coffee or actually seen in the operating room.

This may sound familiar to you as you choose, or have chosen, physicians to manage your care. How, then, do we make these life changing decisions about cancer treatment, in such a brief time, yet in an informed way?

I offer a few specific suggestions?

Turn to knowledgeable people for referrals.

Open yourself up to the possibilities around you. There are people, good people, who want to help. Some care about your family. Some are just good folks. Referrals may come from family, friends, friends of friends, a trusted physician, cancer care specialists, or your local cancer services system. This is called *networking,* something we naturally do when researching schools for our children, looking for jobs, or shopping for a quality used car.

Those who help us locate excellent care do not have to be our best friends. They simply have to be well-informed, credible sources.

Remember, accepting a referral does not in any way obligate us to select the physician or facility that was recommended. The final decisions about treatment are in your hands. These days, when time allows, seeking multiple consultations is a common standard of care.

Allow knowledgeable people to help you access medical care more quickly and personally.

I live close to a metropolitan area rich with excellent medical professionals. Yet, I had no idea how to quickly access the resources specific to my type of cancer, a story have I heard from fellow survivors. And so, with DiAnne by my side, I took another leap of faith, turning to our support system for assistance. Other, more informed people helped me steer a course through the complexities of a large metropolitan teaching hospital. This type of support may also be available to you.

Consider the factors that are most meaningful to you as you choose the medical team.

Decisions about physician choice can are highly personal. I remember someone telling me that when I consulted with surgeons I might find them "less than warm and fuzzy." My response was, "I don't need a surgeon who becomes my friend. I have great friends. I need someone with great skills, someone who listens and answers my questions."

This is exactly what I found, and more, in Dr. Haughey. Once I received his name as a referral, DiAnne and I researched his credentials on the Internet and found an impressive resume, along with numerous powerful, unsolicited testimonials from past patients. However, it was our personal contact with this man that made all the difference. I specifically remember what convinced me that surgery was the correct course of action and that he was the doctor most qualified to meet my needs.

First, Dr. Haughey was the third physician who had scoped my throat and, by far, he had the steadiest hands, gently moving the thin black bendable fiber-optic camera up through my sinus cavity and down to my throat. He then gave me a clear and understandable description of the three recognized treatment approaches for my type and stage of cancer, and why he believed his approach provided the best prognosis. Every question we asked was answered thoroughly and with confidence. He also gave me optimistic, and realistic, data about my chances of recovery. Last, and of great importance, this doctor's approach convinced DiAnne, my number one advocate and most trusted life consultant that he was the right guy for the task at hand. I will never forget his response to her question about prognosis. It went something like this:

Doctor: So, we'll deal with this and in three years we'll get together and share a diet soda.

DiAnne: How about Dom Pierignon?

Doctor: (Smile). OK.

Now, I don't think the good doctor even drinks alcohol. These days, I don't even drink much diet soda, mostly water and juice. It wasn't the words that captured my attention. What mattered was the hope that we derived from his response. Both DiAnne and I left with confidence in the surgical team and a clear message to the doctor's assistant that we wanted my surgery to be scheduled at the earliest possible date.

More than one opinion can make a difference.

What next? Having scheduled my surgery after meeting only one physician, I began the process of choosing radiation and medical oncologists. In my somewhat urgent desire to have a plan, I was tempted to choose the first duo of physicians I met. I took a few deep breaths, knowing that I had several weeks until my surgery. I also took this brief time to research the newest developments in radiation, which helped me make an informed choice.

As a testimony to both my reliance on experts for referrals and my need for empowerment and independence, I met with the oncologists recommended by Dr. Haughey and another physician suggested by a friend. I had some discomfort with both options. One would require significant travel during the advanced stages of my treatment. The other was a fine doctor who was unknown to my surgical team.

At the encouragement of my wife, I scheduled a third consult with a doctor DiAnne was acquainted with. This doctor was affiliated with the city hospital where I would have my surgery, but she was located in a smaller clinic much closer to home. Having grown up in rural communities, I am still most comfortable living in quiet neighborhoods, frequenting a few favorite restaurants and avoiding large parking ramps. I also was deeply concerned about commuting into the city for daily radiation and weekly chemotherapy in terms of time and fatigue. Once again, I can specifically tell you how I knew this third choice was the right place and the right doctor.

I vividly remember the day I first met Dr. Lannis Hall, MD, MPH. I parked a few yards from the front door of the clinic. We walked in and were immediately greeted by the reception staff with a warmth and friendliness that would be reflected in team members throughout the facility. Our wait was short and every professional was kind and thorough. We quickly learned that this clinic used the most up-to-date technology and tools for the treatment of my cancer.

But, once again, the decision was truly made when we met with the doctor. It was the calm confidence and sensitive manner of Dr. Hall that convinced DiAnne and me that we had found another member of our team. She explained her recommendations, answered our questions, heard our fears and actually showed me films that specifically noted where the radiation would be directed on my neck and throat. The doctor was honest and realistic, yet positive. And she listened.

I received further confirmation on meeting Dr. Timothy Pluard, MD, the medical oncologist who was clearly more than an excellent physician. He also listened, provided me with a state-of-the-art chemotherapy plan and took time to answer all of my questions.

One additional factor had a huge impact on my choice. In each previous physician consultation, DiAnne and I expressed concern about my nutrition during recovery. At this clinic, within minutes of presenting our request for information, we met with Leah, the nutritionist whose energy, encouragement, supplements and recipes would be pivotal in my journey through cancer.

This visit affirmed I could get my physical needs met at the local clinic. I felt a stronger sense of hope and confidence knowing that I would be treated by talented, compassionate people in a setting close to home. It would be an exaggeration to say my spirit soared that day, but I was able to smile, cry a bit and tell DiAnne, "This is the place."

What factors are essential to your choices regarding physicians? Experience? Specialization? Education? Accessibility? Bedside manner? Willingness to take time and answer questions? Recommendations from other professionals, family or friends? What are your special needs regarding facilities? State-of-the-art technology and equipment? Accessibility and travel? Insurance and financial issues?

What other services will you need? Nutrition? Support groups? Social Services? Transportation? Relaxation and meditation? Massage therapy? Education regarding side effects, coping with physical changes, dealing with stress, or other emotional concerns? Referrals for financial, social, emotional, or spiritual issues?

Will the facilities you chose either provide you with these services or help you access them from another resource?

Take the time that is realistically and safely available and consider what medical team and facility issues are most important on your path to healing.

A Few More Thoughts on the Challenges of Building a Team

Some survivors and family members face additional complications in selecting treatment providers and in making other early treatment decisions. Perhaps you live in a rural area with more limited hospital and specialty medical services. You may be deciding between a local, narrower range of choices and traveling a significant distance to access more specialized care.

Some of you will be presented with insurance restrictions as you choose providers and facilities. This may be especially true if you receive Medicaid, Medicare, Veterans' benefits, or are uninsured. Finding practitioners who accept your health care plan and understanding exactly what the plan covers will be a crucial aspect of your treatment.

Some of you have a support network that is aging and struggling with their own health issues. You may not have a primary advocate such as a spouse or life partner to rely on through the treatment planning process. You may have language, cultural, or religious concerns that must be addressed, or that may present barriers to getting the treatment you need. Some families face an advanced stage of cancer at the time of diagnosis, requiring immediate decisions about palliative care amidst the shock.

As discussed earlier, some folks have difficulty asking for help, even when significant external obstructions do not exist. Years of working in counseling and addiction services has taught me that fear, shyness, embarrassment and low self-esteem are among the many internal struggles that can greatly interfere with our ability to identify and access necessary resources. I have found this to be most often true among men, but I have certainly known many women who also suffer from self-imposed isolation.

It is vital to transcend this resistance when seeking the best care.

If one or more of the issues above is of concern to you, I suggest you consider the following questions:

> If no one person is available to you as a primary advocate, who do you know among family, friends, acquaintances and community resources who would help you locate doctors and facilities, find transportation, understand your healthcare plan, coordinate financial concerns, and access emotional and spiritual support?
>
> What relationships do you have that could provide support but would require a greater level of cooperation or intimacy than you and this person have enjoyed in the past?
>
> Who will, at the very least, listen and help you to clarify what you want and need to do to obtain the best care available?
>
> Who can help you locate additional community resources?

I had difficulty locating and contacting each and every resource on my own, especially in the days immediately following surgery and in the later stages of radiation and chemo. At every turn, my family and I met people who answered a question or provided a service necessary in that moment. The American Cancer Society, the Council for Aging, The Wellness Community, The United Way, home health agencies, hospital and clinic social workers, insurance company case managers, therapists who specialize in chronic illnesses, local senior centers, local cancer treatment centers and support agencies, national cancer organizations and churches are just some of the concerned groups that create a network of caring to assist us at diagnosis, during treatment, or even in the long term recovery process.

Let yourself be someone who reaches out.

Working with Your Medical Team: Collaboration and Communication

"Most throat cancer survivors get a stomach tube for nutrition. Surgery will disrupt your swallowing reflex. You would have to relearn how to swallow between surgery and starting radiation."

"I'll do whatever I need to."

This was the recommendation of my medical team, followed by my decision not to get a second surgery to insert the tube. I chose to work with a speech pathologist, relearn to swallow and go on a liquid diet for the entire course of therapy. In return for my physicians' willingness to work within my request was my commitment to allow close monitoring of my weight and calorie intake. I also accepted the risk of interrupting treatment if I fell to an unsafe weight and needed the stomach tube.

There would be days as I struggled to consume enough liquid nutrition to sustain myself that I would question my choice. Had I just been stubborn? Should I have gone the other way? Today, I don't believe so. It was a challenge for the whole team and I benefitted from the support of my nutritionist, DiAnne, several close friends and my own persistence to carry on.

It was a group effort.

More than a Survivor: You are a Member of the Team

I had wonderful cancer care. At each stage of my journey, I met highly skilled, efficient and compassionate caregivers.

Not always. At each stage of my journey, I also experienced a smaller number of less skilled, less efficient, grouchy caregivers. I know my experience is not unique.

In most treatment situations, I listened to the advice of the professional caregivers and followed their lead.

Not always. At times, it was necessary to remind myself that I was not just a recipient of care. I was an active, vibrant member of the team that was attempting to restore me to health. After research and consultation, I asked my care system to support several choices that I believed were unique to me and in my best interests. I have heard similar stories from other survivors.

Cancer taught me that it was possible to work cooperatively with most of my treatment staff, while maintaining a realistic level of independence and control. I encourage you to strike this balance whenever possible.

Working Together

One of the early care decisions, made with the input of my wife, was that we would choose doctors and facilities we trusted and then approach them as partners, not adversaries or all-knowing beings.

My job as a cancer survivor (and it has been hard work) included asking questions and gathering as much information as I needed to prepare for each phase of treatment. It also was necessary to open myself to all the resources at hand to combat my disease: medical, physical, emotional and spiritual. I then had to follow through with my commitment to treatment and self-care, even on those most difficult and painful days of my recovery. I struggled, and there were moments when I wanted to give up. It took all of my efforts and the encouragement of many to carry on.

This message is in no way intended to discount your fear of the journey ahead, nor to manufacture some pie-in-the-sky, false optimism. Rather, this is a call to battle. My hope is that you will actively use all of the internal and external resources available to combat your cancer.

Passive compliance, silent resistance, or harsh confrontations with staff will not serve our purposes. We each must find methods for asking questions, engaging our caregivers and challenging unacceptable care, in a way that builds positive working relationships and focuses on problem resolution. At times, this may be exceedingly difficult in the midst of pain, fatigue and fear.

Developing a more personal connection with caregivers and advocates will not be without challenge; it will include cooperation, problem solving and conflict resolution. This is not a bad thing. It is simply the nature of important relationships.

Attitude Counts

Each day when I arrived at the clinic for radiation or chemotherapy, I was greeted by the smile and kind words of Tracy.

Next week, when I go in for my scheduled check-up, I'm sure she, and the other staff I encounter, will smile and tell me how good it is to see me. They care about the patients, about the families, about their work.

As you move through your journey, you will have the opportunity to draw on the energy of people who are compassionate, skilled, optimistic, thorough and available. The most talented caregivers not only provide you with optimum physical care, they help elevate your spirits, restore hope and renew determination.

This was certainly true in my work with Leah, my nutritionist. Throughout treatment, Leah would stop by to offer encouragement and practical solutions. We monitored my calorie intake and weight loss. Each time I tired of my liquid diet, she was there to supply a new recipe, or different calorie and vitamin supplements. She was a coach, a cheerleader and a constant source of information. What was my role? I listened, kept her updated and drank a river of smoothies. This allowed me to maintain a safe weight and not interrupt my treatment.

Attitude counts. This does not mean we have to greet every day with a sunny disposition or mask our true feelings about our pain. I certainly did not. In fact, many of our most valued advocates are intensely interested in honest reports of our symptoms, side effects and shifts in mood.

The mindset I recommend is viewing the support system of professionals, family, friends and other advocates as *your* team. Utilize their skills, communicate as clearly and honestly as your condition allows, give respect, and expect it in return.

And remember, staff are people, too.

Staff are People, Too

Long before the medical staff became the medical staff, each was a person, with dreams and fears and successes and challenges. The staff is not "them." They are just plain folks like us, if we had really cool lab coats.

Dr. Bernie Siegel, the surgeon and amazing author, has devoted decades to the emotional and spiritual aspects of surviving cancer treatment and returning to health.

One of Bernie's ideas stuck to me like glue and made a huge difference in my interactions with the hospital and clinic staff. It went something like:

When I go in for treatment today, I will thank the staff and remember that each of them is a person who left their homes and families on this day to assist me in my recovery.

As I grounded myself in Bernie's suggestion, I became even more aware of the people caring for me and more attuned to the quality of our interactions. I began to use the word "my" not "the" when I discussed surgeons, oncologists and nurses. As this shift occurred, my awareness of the quality of care I was receiving increased. I also realized over a period of months that several of the people providing me services were themselves cancer survivors. Other staff had loved ones who were cancer patients. They, like me, had lived inside this disease. I was filled with gratitude that these people had dedicated their careers to this cause.

And so, sincerely and often, I thanked the staff, from the receptionists to Sue in the billing office to the treatment staff. This was the easiest part of my recovery. I'd met a whole bunch of dedicated, compassionate people.

How might this approach affect our care? I truly believe that seeing the professional team in this light increases our motivation to follow through with even the most challenging aspects of treatment. With collaboration comes the communication that helps prevent errors, promotes quick response to our concerns, bolsters our hope and corrects problems.

When Conflicts Occur: Mutual Respect and Quality Care

As I regained a bit of post-surgery lucidity, I noticed how the hospital staff responded to my wife and how this affected my care. It is not an exaggeration to say that DiAnne is both one of the most personable and most persistent humans on the planet. You may or may not have the miracle of a DiAnne in your life. However, with a few tools your caregivers can provide the advocacy you need during the rigors of treatment.

Looking back, I know that during my hospitalization, good things often happened because she consistently interacted with each staff person from a place I call *respect* and *expect*: I *respect* you as a person and professional and I *expect* you to provide my loved one with excellent care. I watched DiAnne and my sister-in-law, Marilyn, engage tired or distracted staff, not confront or berate them. I saw unit staff, fatigued amidst the incredible demands of the ICU and medical floors, come into my room a bit grumpy and leave with a smile and a kind word. I listened as my advocates respectfully asked questions until we got answers, and firmly but quietly questioned procedures and methods that seemed incongruent with the recovery plan given to us by my surgical team.

And I directly benefited from both of them functioning as members of the team. They made the staff's job a bit easier by making me more comfortable, supervising my erratic behavior in early recovery, helping me get mobile again and facilitating communication between the nursing staff and me as I struggled through the fog.

This was the approach I then adopted for the outpatient portion of my therapy, as I once again became more physically active in my care plan. I viewed the staff as experts and consultants working by my side, not magicians who would cure me or fail me, not impersonal tools to be used simply to meet my needs. I listened, asked questions, disagreed when necessary and, as emphatically as my energy allowed, complied with the plan we designed.

While moving through treatment, you may at times find these ideas very challenging to enact. Fatigue, frustration and worry may affect how you communicate. Perhaps you are an introverted person who finds it difficult to speak openly or disagree with people you see as authorities. You may struggle from the other extreme, tending toward anger and confrontation when confused, worried, or frustrated. Maybe you will encounter people on your medical team who are much less responsive than you require.

It's OK. This plan is not about being perfect. It is about opening your heart to new solutions because…you're not alone.

Addiction as a Key Factor in Treatment Planning

Some survivors will need support services to deal with addictions or compulsive behaviors that could substantially impact success in cancer treatment. Perhaps you have struggled with alcohol or other chemical abuse, smoking, compulsive overeating, or under eating. Planning for these issues is critical to your recovery. Your ability to follow through with the best treatment available, benefit fully from this care, and cope emotionally with both diagnosis and treatment can be directly linked to a program of addiction management and recovery. Further, the safety and success of your cancer care regimen can be significantly affected by hidden, continued addictive behaviors.

Here are a few suggestions:

Be honest with treatment providers about your history of substance use, substance abuse or other health related addictions.

Access information on addiction and cancer care from resources such as the National Cancer Institute.

If you are involved in a program of addiction recovery, such as a 12 Step program, open the door to this support system as part of your cancer care.

If you are not involved in a program of recovery, request information on addiction treatment options as part of your cancer care.

Communicate with your team about any physical and emotional concerns related to your addiction and your cancer care.

In coping with addictions, as with each aspect of the plan, remember that you are not alone.

A Few More Suggestions on Communication

Once again, for successful treatment to take place, survivors and their advocates must have productive ways to communicate with staff. At times, this is easier said than done. Early in the journey, we may be asking questions and receiving instructions through a cloud of fear, confusion and medication. Anger at our disease, or the people involved in our care, may enter the equation. Age, language barriers, family, social and cultural issues also affect how we communicate with words and behavior. The staff, in turn, will vary in skill and compassion, providing care in a high stress environment, responding to a high level of patient need.

I would like to offer a few more specific suggestions that were particularly helpful to me as I waded through the volume of technical information, treatment recommendations and emotions that commanded my attention:

Practice asking caregivers for their time and patience when you are struggling, even when they are busy. Don't assume that others will know when you are confused or hurting. It's OK to gently and firmly insist that others respond to your concerns.

Be assertive in asking for what you need, and then be patient if others occasionally respond in a less than joyful manner. This does not mean you should tolerate rude behavior or incomplete care; remember *respecting* caregivers and *expecting* quality often go hand-in-hand.

Ask for help when experiencing small difficulties, before they became large problems. Keep the important people updated on your progress and on your concerns. Don't wait for a crisis to develop before communicating your struggles, even in the post-treatment stage of recovery.

Ask any question you have about your care. Every question is a good question.

Ask the same question multiple times if the answer is not clear to you. It's possible to listen closely, but still not understand.

Learn the style by which you best grasp important information from staff and advocates. This may include verbal instructions, written word, demonstration and hands-on practice (such as using equipment), and visual aids (such as viewing x-rays). Request information be presented in the style that works best for you.

Allow family and other advocates to ask questions. It is not necessary for you to think of every question or remember every answer.

Ask that instructions on self-care to be repeated until both you and your closest advocates understand each procedure.

Empower trusted family and friends to speak on your behalf when you are unable (post-surgery, medical crisis).

Respectfully confront staff when you are provided with inadequate information, incorrect or incomplete care. Empower trusted family and friends to do the same if you are unable to clearly communicate.

And when you are able, thank your best caregivers for exceptional and compassionate assistance.

A Special Message of Encouragement for Men

As I move through the world of aftercare, cancer prevention and cancer research, I am amazed and impressed by the organized presence of breast cancer survivors. I have asked myself how this particular group of fellow travelers has created such a powerful voice amongst the multitude of survivors.

I don't know for sure, but as a therapist with years of specializing in men's issues and gender concerns, this is my theory:

One aspect of visibility and advocacy among breast cancer survivors is that the majority (95 percent) are female. Women, in general, value relationship and emotional support to a degree that we men, while hungry for, are often socialized to discount or view in the negative. The openness to connection that pervades the lives of many women helps to promote a system of group support, advocacy for research and dedication to prevention which has spawned a movement. This network provides an incredible community of empathy for the pain, and sometimes loss, that survivors' experience, along with a joyful celebration of life.

As male survivors, we can learn from this. In many ways the idiom "Big Boys Don't Cry" is still alive and well in our world. In my work life I have often responded to this cliché with "But Big Men Do." Whether expressing my concerns during treatment, experiencing the relief and joy of healing moments, or facing the possibility of unwanted outcomes, it has been OK, even essential, to set aside old worn out ideas about masculinity and open my heart to those I most love and trust. Not everyone gets to see the softer side of me…but a few of my most precious advocates do.

When I hear fellow male survivors discuss the value of their support groups for prostate cancer, I am greatly encouraged. When I hear their disappointment that so many of us are unable to push through the extreme sense of vulnerability brought on by our illness and our culture, and so, we remain disconnected from available prevention and support strategies, I am saddened.

Releasing emotional pain can free up energy for the tasks at hand. Independence, emotional honesty and social connections are not mutually exclusive, they are complimentary.

Opening our hearts to a wide web of community and connection also lightens the load for our loved ones, removing the unrealistic expectation that one or two people must shoulder the entire burden of physical and emotional support. Allowing a network of advocates into our lives can allay another fear carried by many families, that we, as men, will simply remain isolated in our pain, forfeiting that crucial fighting spirit.

This issue of disconnection also merits close consideration if you are a male caregiver. Isolation breeds fear, resentment and depression, whether you are in recovery from cancer or assisting a survivor through their journey. This will be especially critical if you have relied in the past on the survivor for most of your emotional sustenance, and are now faced with the role of primary caregiver. The survivor will, at times, need to conserve his or her energy for the work ahead and will be comforted by the knowledge that you will seek input and understanding from other, healthy sources.

Let me assure you that I do not propose this change in a casual way. For some of us, transforming a lifetime of playing our emotional cards close to the vest will come as a hard fought battle. However, desperate times often call for desperate measures. For some of us, these are desperate times.

And so, for men and women, I offer the following affirmation:

Courage comes in many forms. It takes a special daring for us as survivors and caregivers to step beyond our comfort zones, allowing others to not only see our strength, but our vulnerability.

Collaboration: Also More than Physical

"I'm tired."
"I'm scared."
"I'm confused."
"I'm ticked off."
"I'm just glad to be here."

These are words I have repeated to numerous friends and family members in the course of my recovery. In reply, I was given hugs, sympathy, encouragement and the occasional loving confrontation.

The rigors of cancer call upon many of us to connect with internal sources of strength beyond any demanded in previous life challenges. Intangible resources such as hope, motivation, tenacity, determination and faith are powerful allies as we move through pain, progress and setbacks. The quality and depth of our social, physical, emotional and spiritual support system is a circle of life around which we can build, maintain and, in times of loss, rebuild our will to fight.

Hope

Psychiatrist and cancer specialist Dr. David Spiegel has written extensively on the value of social connection in cancer care. His pioneering work in group therapy tells us that emotional support and expressive therapy significantly improve the ability of breast cancer survivors to cope with stress, combat depression and manage pain (Spiegel 1989). He believes that treatment follow-through can be enhanced by the quality of social connection in a survivor's world. In my mind, as a survivor, this translates into a greater chance for healing.

Dr. Spiegel and Dr. Ernest H. Rosenbaum emphasize the value of supportive care in mobilizing us, as survivors, to maintain a sense of control and a positive attitude in the midst of fear, fatigue, pain, feelings of helplessness and the awareness our mortality.

"A fighting spirit, a trusting relationship with the medical team, access to information and support programs, the support of family and friends, the balancing of life and illness, and a strong sense of hope all promoted through a supportive care regimen can enhance the empowerment of cancer patients(Rosenbaum and Spiegel, www.cancersupportivecare.com/empower)."

These experts validate what my heart already knows; personal empowerment and interpersonal support systems are powerful factors in the journey through cancer. By linking arms with medicine, family, friends and other advocates, I was given a fighting chance.

Hope for Family and Friends

Peter R. VanDermoot, founder of the Children's Treehouse Foundation, an organization which provides emotional support to children who have parents with cancer reported that an estimated 315,247 parents of ages 25-54 will be diagnosed with invasive cancer each year, impacting approximately 592,000 children (Howard 2007).

The support system we develop for this journey, the, must also address the need of our children, spouses, partners and other loved ones. The community that gathered around me was available to every individual within the circle.

For some of us, this idea necessitates another shift in belief. A common myth about the risk of reaching out to others in a time of struggle is that we must relinquish our control, our power to make independent decisions. In truth, extending our reach beyond medicine and technology into the social, emotional and spiritual support we need is a recipe for empowerment, both increasing our independence and providing our loved ones with increased options for assisting in our care.

My journey is packed with stories of the mutual care and compassion supplied by one of my advocates to another. They not only took care of me, they took care of one another. This is not an easy task given the number of independent souls that inhabit my world.

How did this happen? A combination of *reality* and *attitude*. The *reality* is that I have cultivated relationships with strong, vibrant, loving people throughout my adult life. This may or may not be your experience. If your reality is a support group that is more limited in size or vitality, the *attitude* of an open heart becomes essential not only to survivors, but to the health of those that provide our care. This means allowing new resources to come into our recovery so those we most count on can, at times, step away and replenish their resources.

Remember, building the most extensive circle of care available allows advocates to share the responsibilities of care giving, a key to their own well-being. As I have continued on the path through cancer, I am acutely aware of the extreme levels of stress, fatigue, fear and frustration placed by this illness on our families and closest friends. Marshalling the full extent of available resources will not only increase our own sense of empowerment, but will also nurture families and friends as they lead and follow us through the days, months and, sometimes, years of recovery.

Caring for Our Caregivers

At times, people who care about me try to protect me from difficult news in their lives, "Chris, I didn't want to worry you, you've been sick". My answer has been to smile and say, "I am aware that while I have been recovering from cancer, the world continues to turn much as before."

My reply has a two-fold meaning. First, I know that each member of a support network experiences daily challenges throughout the time they are assisting in our care. Some of these struggles are related to our health, some are simply the stuff of life. The car still needs a new battery, kids still have homework, the holidays still arrive. Second, cancer does not rob survivors of our abilities to love, empathize, or care about our caregivers. Part of empowerment in this journey is the knowledge that we still have something to give. Offering our end of positive connection is a reminder that giving as well as receiving love can energize us and keep the fires of hope alive.

During treatment I would doggedly pursue my routine with certain family members, asking, "And how was your day?" I would then offer my typically unsolicited opinions on how they could solve certain problems, approach issues of concern, or enjoy the good times. Often I was told, directly or indirectly, "Don't worry about me." In fact, I needed to be concerned about those that I love, and so will you.

It is remarkable to me how many survivors and family members I have met who continue to give extraordinary gifts of physical, emotional and spiritual support to others while in the throes of their cancer journey, each one of them digging deep to provide support to family, friends and strangers who became friends. Cancer does not define us. We are survivors, caregivers, and much, much more.

How will continuing to actively participate in the lives of family and friends increase your quality of life?

What about Our Children?

Many of us will be actively engaged in parenting throughout treatment and recovery. We may still be raising young folks. We may have adult children who are involved in our care and deeply impacted by our illness. The effects on children of all ages who have a parent, or parents, struggling with cancer are substantial. Yet, this disease can also offer incredible opportunities to strengthen bonds that already exist between parents and children.

DiAnne and I chose to wait a few days, until we had the basics of a treatment plan, before telling our children of my diagnosis. This gave us time to prepare how we would explain my situation and time to prepare for their response. Our children were all old enough to understand the possible implications of cancer, able to ask specific and detailed questions, and able to do their own research.

Your circumstances might be very different from mine. A variety of factors will determine your child's reaction to this news; age, stage of development, personality, and the quality of the relationship are several key aspects for consideration. How you communicate with your child also will be affected by your prognosis and the anticipated impact of your treatment on the family. Take the time to seek counsel and prepare yourself to discuss your diagnosis with your kids in a way that considers their needs.

Cancer served as another reminder in my life that each of my children is a unique individual; they had distinct styles of coping with my illness over the long term. At different times I heard sympathy, humor, silence, encouragement and loving confrontation.

There have been moments along this road when I have been deeply concerned about the strain placed on my children as they worked, went to school and coped with their daily stress, all the while supporting me through therapy and recovery.

Our children are not simply witnesses to these events; they are a part of the team.

And so, one essential aspect of treatment is gathering resources to meet the special needs of our children. Many clinics now provide outstanding support options for helping children manage the disruption that cancer brings. Treatment centers often offer playgroups for younger kids and support services to children of parents in treatment. Social workers, psychologists and therapists who specialize in health issues provide individual and family therapy to kids in need. Adult family and friends can also provide a heightened level of sensitivity to children who are walking this road with a parent. I have heard more than one wonderful story of a neighborhood coming together to be the village the helps raise the children of survivors in recovery.

Your children will have another incredibly valuable resource: you. Each time I had the opportunity to speak with one of my kids about school or work or the special events in their lives, I became more than a cancer survivor again, for them and for myself. Each time I participated in some aspects of their lives, no matter how small, we experienced moments of normalcy, a reminder to all that our family was much more than my illness.

Children can give us a powerful sense of purpose. I offer what I'm certain is only a partial list of the blessings that can be contributed by young people in our pursuit of recovery:

Optimism and faith: Children often possess an amazing capacity to believe in the best of all possible outcomes.

Trust: Our kids need to trust that we are devoted not only to them, but to our own health and well-being.

Distraction: Caring for our children can be a temporary diversion from the rigors of cancer. To the degree that we are able, participating in the daily events of family life provides a sense of empowerment, productivity and satisfaction that helps to offset the attention commanded by illness and recovery.

Participation: Children differ in their ability and need to be present during various phases of recovery. This will be affected by age, coping skills and other needs. It is essential not to ask children to participate at a level beyond what is appropriate for their development. It is just as crucial not to shut them out in a misdirected attempt to protect them from the truth of a parent's illness.

Motivation: Watching our children grow can be a potent motivator for staying committed to the best options in self-care. A casual conversation about the school day, or a boyfriend, or the kid who blew milk out of his nose at daycare can put a little gas in a parent's emotional, spiritual and physical tank.

What are the special needs of the children in your life with regard to cancer? Information? Support? The opportunity to help? Whether you are a parent, grandparent, aunt, uncle, or friend, how might you include a child in your community of healing?

A Few Thoughts on Finances

The financial cost of cancer care is, by my standards, enormous. My treatment and aftercare have cost thousands and thousands of dollars, and there will be more. As a private businessman, I was unable to work for a number of months. Our family relied totally on my spouse for financial support during my therapy.

I know my story is not unique. For most of us, the economics of recovery is a priority issue in the journey to health. In my business I deal with insurance companies on a daily basis, and yet, managing the complexities of payment for the various aspects of cancer care was confusing and stressful. My wife was exceptional in helping me coordinate this concern. Even with my knowledge and her efforts, we spent out-of-pocket dollars from our family's budget that could have been saved had we better understood the system.

Whatever your healthcare payment circumstances, I encourage you to access your plan's case coordination structure. All private insurance providers offer services to assist in precertification, explain patient deductibles and copayments, insure that prescribed tests and medications are within the company's payment guidelines, and assist in the submission and payment of claims. Some companies provide case managers for clients dealing with major health issues; this allows you to communicate with the same person on an ongoing basis, someone who is familiar with you and your situation. If you receive other forms of benefits, such as public or Veterans' assistance, locating specific individuals within the provider systems who will assist you in coordinating financial concerns is a crucial portion of your overall care. Some cancer centers even provide navigators, individuals who are specially trained to help survivors and families access necessary services along the entire spectrum of care.

Many of us are uninsured or underinsured. Hospitals and clinics offer social workers who consult on many components of treatment, including financial issues. Some systems provide financial assistance to families who can identify need. Social workers helped me quickly acquire some of the equipment and nutritional aids I needed, at more reasonable costs than I could have found these resources on my own.

At times, treatment settings assist in payment for care, transportation, essential medications and other specialty services. Local cancer agencies also may provide this type of advocacy. For example, in the metropolitan area where I received my surgery, the Wellness Community provides a broad range of free services to meet the educational, psychological and spiritual needs of survivors and families. National services, such as the CancerCare website, offer methods to identify and contact numerous financial resources.

Another major asset in managing the complications of payment was the billing department of my clinic. I was able to speak face-to-face with a knowledgeable, local person who became my advocate in fully utilizing my healthcare benefits.

Once again, all questions are good questions. As survivors and family, we are ultimately responsible for the cost of our treatment, whether we understood our healthcare benefits or not. Even in the best of care systems, we may learn about all financial assistance options only by forming new, working relationships with facility and community resources and by asserting our specific needs. Once again, silence or believing that others should simply know what we need will not serve us well.

Whatever your concerns, take time to speak directly with knowledgeable people at your insurance company or other healthcare benefit organization. Request a consultation with the hospital and clinic social work departments to discuss your special financial needs and available services. Contact your local cancer society and other reputable cancer support systems to learn of economic supports for survivors and families.

Again, let yourself be someone who asks for help.

TREATMENT AND RECOVERY

"Last year when my wife was re-diagnosed, our friends put together a surprise trivia night fundraiser. It was the weekend before her birthday, so we celebrated that too! There were over 400 people there. It was incredibly touching that they decided to do this so she could focus on treatment."

Caregiver

Hospital Care

"Time for a walk down the hall."
"I don't really feel like it."
"Let's go, honey."
"OK. You're tough."

Sometimes, objective professional staff will be most powerful in motivating us to participate fully in our hospital care. At other moments our personal support system will be instrumental in our movement to the next level of recovery. The cooperation of all team members gives us the best possible of results.

Family Centered Care

Through cancer, I learned that one essential measure of the quality of care I will receive during any hospital admission goes beyond the technology and expertise of the staff: it includes the facility's policy on family and patient participation in patient care.

The most advanced cancer treatment centers see loved ones as assets in the recovery process, rather than impediments to getting the job done. The best surgeons bring family into the communication loop. For example, during my nine-plus hours of surgery my wife was given several updates on my progress. Post-surgery, we were able to arrange for family to be present on a twenty-four hour basis throughout my hospital stay. Forward-thinking medical facilities know that the pace and demands of patient care on nursing staff have significantly accelerated in our current healthcare environment. They welcome the positive participation of personal caregivers.

Without my family's help during the initial days of my recovery, my confusion may have caused me to pull life-preserving tubes out of my body. I may have languished in bed when I needed to become mobile. Family helped me interpret certain self-care instructions. They prevented several potential medical errors when the doctor's orders were not completely clear to the nursing staff and I could not communicate my concerns.

After surgery, I could not swallow and so I could not lie down. As I sat in my chair, DiAnne helped me catch snippets of sleep. Marilyn stayed with me for an entire night, so DiAnne could get a few hours sleep. They both listened to my fears, confusion and frustration until the Chris they were familiar with began to reappear. These are functions that nursing staff cannot perform. For this we need other advocates.

My personal support system also helped save considerable time and effort for me and the unit staff: they helped me stand and walk, monitored my pain, and met basic needs of warmth and liquids. They challenged me to follow the daily plan so I could go home.

In short: family, friends and other caregivers can be present and actively engaged during our hospital stays, until we are lucid and mobile enough to more fully participate in our own care.

During my hospital stay I also became a member of the team. On several occasions, as my thinking began to clear, I fostered communication between the physicians and nursing staff, ensuring they clarify discrepancies in my plan.

Family-centered care will positively impact your return to health. Make it a common goal for all caregivers.

Using All of Your Resources

"We'll be getting to know one another pretty well. We'll get through this together."

These kind words came from a fine young man, Dr. Allen, who followed me in my first days post-surgery. Many thousands of patients from now I doubt that he will have any memory of me. But, DiAnne and I will never forget his compassionate care.

I believe in my heart and soul that the quality connections I had with professionals, friends and especially family carried me through those most taxing months of treatment. This is a message I carry to you.

Doctors, Nurses and More

As we enter treatment, we learn that physicians and nursing staff are only the beginning of the professionals who can and will assist us in our recovery. Other professionals that had a major impact on my journey, included:

Hospital: Medical supply staff, pharmacists, lab technicians, pulmonary techs, nutritionists, home health coordinators, emergency room staff

Hospital-based outpatient clinic: Speech pathologists

Outpatient care: Radiation technologists, physician's assistants, nurse practitioners, nursing assistants, physicists, billing staff, nutritionists, a massage therapist, social workers, lab staff, pharmacists, PET and CAT scan technologists, reception and scheduling staff

Community services: home health, social services, pastoral care, local cancer society, medical supply

Be sure to familiarize yourself with the full range of services offered by the hospitals and clinics that you are engaging for treatment. Let the social work staff help you identify and contact community resources for counseling, transportation, medical supply, childcare and other support options.

Even if you and family members do extensive research on your particular cancer care needs, ask the professional staff about additional services that will help you heal. For example, massage therapy has been extremely useful as I cope with the effects of surgery and radiation on my neck and shoulders.

Managing Side Effects: Also More than Physical

The side effects of cancer medication and therapy are diverse and serious. Excellent communication with staff and other caregivers is one key to managing this portion of our struggle. Once again, silent suffering or complaining without a plan will not do.

Among the numerous side effects I dealt with during treatment, my most difficult included nausea, dehydration, a painful skin rash and my intense anxiety regarding radiation. In each case, collaboration with my medical team and other allies eased the struggle. By staying in close contact with Dr. Pluard and Donna's infusion team, we were able to react quickly to my dehydration and not interrupt the schedule of treatment. I owe so much to the rapid response of this group of care providers. Likewise, Viki, my nurse practitioner, monitored and helped me manage a rash that was frustrating, very painful and embarrassing.

I remember one simple example that highlights the importance of close contact with the team. As I began chemotherapy, I was continuing to have some difficulty swallowing. The nurses asked me if I could swallow pills before treatment and I said "yes." I did not realize the pill they had in mind was dry, with no coating to make it go down more easily. Rather than express my concern I got the medication down in the first week of therapy. Not so the following week, when attempting to swallow the medication stimulated my extremely active gag reflex. Not a pretty sight.

This episode clearly communicated to the nurses what I had failed to put into words. For future treatments they gave me the same med in liquid form. What was the lesson? I was trying to be unnecessarily cooperative and strong. But, the nurses who were just getting to know me were counting on an honest answer to their question as a guide to planning.

Not all of my issues with side effects were so easily resolved. At times, I learned that all that could be done to assist me was already being done. While frustrating, it helped a bit to know we were all already doing the best we could.

By keeping the staff updated on my progress, condition and concerns, we were able to minimize, even prevent, a number of other treatment crises. I encourage each of you to respond honestly to questions from the team about your condition and to be proactive; offer unsolicited information and questions about the effects of therapy. Become an active member in developing a recovery plan that evolves and reacts to your current circumstance.

Not all side effects are physical. Cancer brings a variety of emotional responses, many of which may deepen as we travel further into treatment. Our feelings can develop into depression and anxiety, both of which are greatly under-reported and under-diagnosed in survivors. Some survivors have struggled with these concerns prior to any cancer diagnosis. Some of us will experience previously unknown emotional challenges directly connected to diagnosis and treatment.

Our emotions also can bring us to spiritual crisis, struggling with the seeming unfairness of this illness, with anger at God, or even with questions about the very purpose of life. There is also help for these difficulties.

For example, as an oral cancer patient I found the process of radiation particularly anxiety producing. The emotional challenge of radiation was, at first, initially much more difficult than the physical. Although I am not claustrophobic, I became very fearful when my mobility was restricted during the initial treatments. I am indebted to a number of people for assisting me through this trial.

By communicating my discomfort to the radiation team, I received detailed information on how I would be made as comfortable as possible, along with the team's patience and compassion. Then, my wonderful and talented friend Jim helped me design a guided imagery that I used as relaxation therapy, bringing me comfort and taking the edge off of my fears. Each day when I lay on the table I focused on this reassuring and healing imagery. Finally, I was lovingly challenged by my wife and my business partner Mark to utilize the medication offered by the doctor to help manage my anxiety.

Remember, the rigors of treatment can trigger fear, anger, guilt and sadness. These feelings can evolve into painful conditions that can significantly hamper our follow through and response to the recovery plan. Excellent help is available for our emotional and spiritual struggles, just as state-of-the-art technology addresses our physical healing.

Here are a few tools to for this part of your journey:

Continue to ask yourself if you are frustrated, fearful, embarrassed, sad, or guilty about your cancer, or the limitations it brings into your life.

Be honest and open with advocates about the emotional side effects of cancer and treatment. Remember, it takes a special strength, not weakness, to discuss emotional concerns.

Stay as physically active as your illness allows. We know that physical activity supports a positive mood and enhances that ever important fighting spirit. As the good doctor, Dr. Haughey, told me in the advanced stages of my healing, "Keep exercising. Don't favor yourself so much."

Use your staff nutritionist to help maintain energy, strength and mood stability.

Use the support network provided by your hospital and clinic: social services, support groups, informational sessions and wellness workshops.

Allow yourself to turn to professional resources such as counseling and medications for depression and anxiety. These services can greatly enhance your motivation, optimism and willingness to follow the plan.

Communicate spiritual and religious concerns to trusted, nonjudgmental advocates. Let go of any guilt or shame you may feel when experiencing doubt, frustration or fear, even if you are a deeply devout person. We are human. Healthy spiritual support does not require constant and absolute faith.

Remember, we are mind, body and spirit. A comprehensive strategy for coping with the effects of treatment will fortify us and greatly enhance our quality of life.

There are No Strangers in Foxholes: Allow Help to Find You

"There are no strangers in foxholes" is an adaptation of a religious saying. I probably first heard this modification from one of my dad's friends—perhaps a war veteran. In a few words, this powerful truth tells me that relationship bonds can be formed quickly, for very specific reasons, in the heat of battle.

Webster's Dictionary offers the first-line definition that a friend is "a person whom one knows well and is fond of (Webster's New World Dictionary, 2003)." This certainly fits the way I have characterized friendship over most of my life. However, a bit further down the page, the good folks at Webster's expand the meaning of friend to include a slightly different interpretation that offers a profound opportunity for us as cancer survivors. A friend also is "an ally, supporter, or sympathizer (Webster's New World Dictionary, 2003)."

In this second description, how well one knows an ally may not be of primary concern. What matters is the existence of meaningful support. The immediacy of crisis sometimes calls upon us to suspend the usual time requirements for getting acquainted, to open our hearts as opportunity knocks. I have vigorously applied this idea in pursuit of healing.

I hope you have cultivated a strong circle of friendship that can be easily accessed for physical, emotional and spiritual backup. If you have drifted away from old friends, this is a time for reconnection. You may need to push through your reluctance to asking for what you need from familiar pals and loved ones.

New friends and advocates also will appear. Some connections will be brief. Other people will come into your world and remain as important members of the recovery team.

Certain folks will arrive, provide just the right support at just the right time, and then be gone.

I met the same two gentlemen in the radiation therapy waiting room on numerous occasions, one who received treatment before me and one who followed right after. We'd exchange pleasantries, compare symptoms and side effects, and discuss how we were managing in our daily lives. Although I never saw these men outside the clinic, we developed a unique intimacy, disclosing very personal fears and frustrations in graphic language. I have facilitated a lot of group therapy over the years. Several of my closest male friends come from a men's support group I belonged to for more than a decade. Still, I have never experienced anything quite like this makeshift group, crafted by three strangers, squeezed into a few minutes time frame, with no particular plan beyond, "how ya doin' today?" These opportunities will be presented to you.

Other additions to your support network may involve allies who have only been on the periphery of your life before cancer. I was deeply touched by the friend of a friend who I had met through my work some years previous. This gentleman, who I barely knew, had received the same diagnosis as mine, was several months further into his treatment process, and called me to offer his support. On several occasions, once on very short notice, he arrived with words of encouragement and concrete information about managing the side effects of radiation and chemotherapy. To have the input of a fellow throat cancer survivor was a huge emotional boost.

At times, cancer wants to drive us inward, fostering social and emotional isolation. Fatigue, pain and other stressors can disconnect us from our surroundings, including the efforts of others to reach into our world. It is essential to know that each one of us deserves the gestures of kindness that come our way.

I will always remember John. It seemed that every time I called in an order of my nutrition drink to the medical supply store, he would answer the phone. I began to look forward to seeing him when I went in to pick up a fresh case. He would always take an extra moment to ask me how treatment was proceeding. One day, when I was walking the dog, John jogged past and stopped to check in. After that, I saw him jogging or driving home from work on several more occasions. He always slowed and waved.

Most recently, I stopped into the medical supply store to get a case of the same drink for another survivor. John told me he'd been wondering how I was and that I had been in his prayers. I was a bit overwhelmed.

We won't always know why we are the recipients of these selfless actions. Some folks will choose to share their own stories, some will not. Their motives are not what matters. What counts is our willingness to collect the love and support made available to us in the vigorous pursuit of treatment and recovery.

Active Participation Works, Too

Some of us will prefer to get more into the mix actively create new connections.

Here are a few suggestions for those of you who want to generate a more effective support system:

Attend a cancer survivor program at your clinic or hospital. Workshops and support groups provide practical information, expand awareness of available services and facilitate contact with other survivors and caregivers. These environments exist to send the message "we care and we understand." As previously stated, strong evidence exists that follow-through with care and quality of life are significantly affected by attending survivors support groups.

Attend a cancer survivor event in your community. My email is regularly bombarded with announcements of what's happening in the local and national movements to conquer this disease. If your health limits energy or mobility, I have found that each of us is welcome to attend for whatever time we can manage and to simply rest among those who truly understand. Cancer care functions come in all shapes and sizes: small and large, indoors and outdoors, serious and playful.

Contact a local or national cancer advocacy network. The range of services provided by some of these groups extends far beyond research and fundraising, and is often accessible by phone, email, snail mail, even personal visits. What we will find in the voice at the other end of the phone, the message in our email, or the face of the person knocking on our door is compassion and understanding. In that moment, one person may change our lives.

What resources exist in your community, or are accessible through electronic sources, to create a stronger support system for you and your advocates during the intensity of primary treatment? How do you access this network? How will you access this network?

More Emotional Support: Some Days are Tougher than Others

As my treatment advanced, there were days when I decided I would not get up and go to the clinic. Nathan had left for school, DiAnne for work. I was alone, in bed, frustrated, nauseous and exhausted. I remember saying to myself, "I'm done. I felt better before they started curing me of this [expletive deleted] disease."

Without fail, in those dark moments, the phone would ring. It was usually DiAnne:

"Are you up (her voice holding an amazing combination of loving concern and direct challenge)?"

"Yup (being a genuinely honest person, I'm climbing out of bed as I reply)."

"Putting any calories in?"

"Heading for the refrigerator right now. Going to make another delicious smoothie."

"Well, you're a bit behind on calories for the day already, honey (not falling for the thinly veiled sarcasm)."

"I'll take something with me to drink during treatment."

"Great. Love you. Call me after treatment to tell me how it went."

"Love you. Bye."

Each day, by the end of this conversation, I had re-committed to go to the clinic, drink my calories and get through another treatment. Love can be a tricky thing. In my life, it sometimes involved following through on commitments that were, to put it mildly, extremely unpleasant.

Some of your most loving support will come in the form of challenge, perhaps even compassionate confrontation. You don't need to rely exclusively on your own strength to push through the physical and emotional rigors of treatment. You don't need to always be cheerful, or motivated, or even willing. Some days, the best you can do is to connect with someone who will help you get through the next test, the next procedure, the next side effect.

One step, one meal, one medication, one treatment, one day at a time.

I Have a Good Support System: I'm Still Anxious

I often think of anxiety as the physical manifestation of fear and worry. Racing thoughts, sleeplessness, sweats, heart palpitations, a general sense of foreboding, shortness of breath. If you experience anxiety related to your diagnosis and treatment, making the positive choice to seek additional help can have a considerable impact on your quality of life and treatment follow-through.

Even with the incredible physical and emotional support I was receiving, anxiety was a daily presence for me, from pre-diagnosis to aftercare. Today, as I look toward an upcoming check-up, I still feel a twinge of that old familiar fear.

As mentioned earlier, my anxiety reached an overwhelming level as I entered the radiation phase of treatment. In addition to my physical struggles, I began to feel bad about myself. I had hoped that through my training in relaxation therapy, lots of prayer and the sensitivity of the staff, I could manage. Some days I couldn't. My anxiety ranged from relative calm to edginess to periods of near panic.

For me, the answer included medication. Counselors, loved ones, guided imagery, medications. All of these resources are at our disposal to comfort and assist us through each stage of therapy, improving the process of the treatment itself and our quality of life when we are not in the treatment room.

Courage, willpower, inner strength and faith are all admirable. Sometimes, they are enough. Sometimes, we waver. This is not bad. This is normal.

Be honest with yourself. Be honest with your caregivers. Call upon all the resources available to cope with fear, worry and anxiety.

Depression: What to Do When You're More than Blue

Even the most optimistic, engaged and courageous among us can experience a depressed mood, irritability, loss of interest in daily activities, and crying spells as therapy advances. Chemotherapy, radiation and pain medications combine with the wide range of stressors that cancer often brings. This may result in poor concentration, sleeplessness, poor appetite, decreased libido, emotional and social withdrawal.

Feelings of helplessness and hopelessness are of special concern and must be addressed as part of our recovery. Managing the physical demands of therapy alongside even a mild depression can be increasingly difficult.

Once again, by seeking help for the emotional aspects of the cancer journey, you can greatly enhance your quality of life and full participation in the healing process.

Your family and the peer support system you have developed can provide significant relief from the strong emotional and physical changes that can morph into depression. For some of us, staying in close contact with loved ones will be enough to see us through.

Some of us will benefit greatly from professional intervention. Cancer treatment centers are increasingly aware of the prevalence and treatment of the depression that can occur at any phase of the recovery process, from diagnosis through aftercare. Support groups, individual counseling and anti-depressant medications are all options for survivors in need.

As always, the healing begins with us. You don't need to completely understand the differences between cancer's side effects, anxiety and depression to investigate a change in emotions or mood. Discuss your concerns. Access information on the connection between cancer and depression. Work with the medical staff to identify mood changes, determine what the symptoms mean and design a plan for intervention.

The Importance of Healing Touch

I remember reading the statement of a cancer survivor who was a member of Congress. He spoke eloquently of the sense that some people treated him as if he had a contagious disease, fearful of direct contact.

For many of us, cancer impacts our physical appearance, self-esteem and social interactions. How can others help us manage the more intangible effects of these changes?

I can tell you exactly how this works. In every phase of my cancer journey, I have had professionals who will look at me, speak directly with me about every confusing or embarrassing aspect of my illness, and treat me as more than a cancer survivor. One of my favorite caregivers is a massage therapist who combines healing touch with listening to my story, and telling her own.

In every phase of my cancer journey, I also have had family and friends who would look me in the eye and touch me. Loved ones touched my hand, put suave on a rash I could not reach, washed my hair when I could not lift my arms, helped me get dressed when my coordination was somewhat less than that an Olympic gymnast. They laughed along with the dark humor I occasionally found necessary to cope with radiation tattoos, regression to adolescent acne and the fear that comes with a Stage 4 diagnosis. They held me when I cried. They hugged me when the news was scary. They hugged me when the news was joyful. They all touched me. Not just emotionally and spiritually, but literally.

Whether you need a hug or a kiss, to be held when in pain, or a fist bump when you receive wonderful news, reach out to those who aren't afraid to connect. Physical affection, comforting touch, massage, sexual intimacy with your spouse or life partner; these are all crucial to our well-being and quality of life. Some people will just know. Other times, we need to communicate our desires. This, too, calls for collaboration and cooperation.

And remember, when you allow yourself the blessing of healing touch, you also touch the life of the healer.

Each Journey is a Work in Progress

"I'm not feeling well. I'm not sure I can make it in for treatment today."

"Can you come in right now? We'll see what we can do."

This phone call took place more than once in the later stage of primary treatment. I was fortunate that the team could respond to my struggles. Some interventions worked better than others. From the evolution of my treatment, however, I learned a valuable lesson that I have seen countless times since, in the recovery of fellow survivors.

The first plan is often not the last plan.

The Science and Art of Survivorship

I had a treatment plan. So will you. The plan was specific, based on the current research and state-of-the-art technology.

The plan also evolved as my needs and response to therapy changed, based on the experience, finest ideas and instincts of the best caregivers I could find. I would have preferred absolute certainty and a 100 percent positive, won't-need-money-back, guarantee. What I got was the experience, finest ideas and instincts of the best caregivers I could find.

Much is known about cancer care. Much is yet to be known. Cancer care experts know a great deal about how we as survivors will respond to certain forms of surgery, radiation, chemo and other medications. Yet the effectiveness and affects of various strategies are unique to individual survivors, and cannot always be known until treatment is initiated.

A common side effect of the chemo I received is a skin condition similar to acne, but more painful and covering a lot more territory on the body. No one could know that I would have a severe reaction until therapy progressed. For me, the impact was both physical and emotional: significant discomfort and a change in appearance that I could see every morning in the mirror, one that has left marks of reminder about my treatment.

My medical team had several options to assist me physically. Various medications eased the discomfort and allowed me to continue chemo uninterrupted by this condition. None of them worked particularly well, from my perspective. They just allowed us to go forward.

This is a small example of the importance of flexibility in the plan for recovery. Many of us will need more significant adaptations in our therapy. Based on the success of certain treatments, the type and stage of your cancer, and almost constant advances in the field, science and art must combine as we work together to creatively address this complex illness.

As with diagnosis and initial planning, the progression of medical treatment calls on each component of our support system to cope with the successes and set-backs of this evolving road map for recovery. As we collaborate with medical staff to maximize our healing and minimize our physical distress, other advocates will help of remain connected with hope and discouragement, faith and fear, understanding and uncertainty.

Primary Treatment, Aftercare and More

The treatment plan for cancer contains lots of numbers: timelines, dosages, numbers of radiation and chemotherapy treatments. At first glance, it would seem to be an exact science. However, we are the human factor and our response to treatment can change the numbers.

For some of us, the numbers are not finite, based on partial remission or an extended course of treatment. Even if active treatment concludes, maintaining gains and monitoring health are ongoing concerns for all survivors and families.

As so, the journey through cancer moves toward ongoing care and aftercare.

AFTERCARE: ONGOING RECOVERY AND THE OPPORTUNITY TO GIVE BACK

"I can spend the day in bed recounting the difficulty I have with the parts of my body that don't work or get out of bed and be thankful for the ones that do. Older age is like a bank account. You withdraw what you put in. My advice would be to deposit a lot of happiness in your bank and…give more."

Survivor quoting a favorite saying

Ongoing Care

"I'll see you next month."

The journey through cancer does not have a specific ending point. I continue to visit regularly with many of the professionals that followed me through primary care. For some of us, treatment will be ongoing. Therapy can be open-ended. A return to treatment is possible for some of us. Even when treatment is completed with optimum outcomes, physical recovery takes time.

The physicality of illness and therapy can have a wide range of enduring effects on survivors, including limited mobility, changes in physical appearance, or any number of other minor to severe to debilitating challenges that require lifestyles adjustments and creative problem-solving.

These variations in healing are just as true for us as emotional and spiritual beings. The social and community resources needed by those of us receiving ongoing medical treatment are different from those of the person whose primary care has a conclusion. Regardless of the path through physical recovery, it takes time, contemplation and conversation to integrate the changes that cancer brings in how we view ourselves, our relationships with others and, in some cases, our spiritual vision.

Because our medical issues as survivors are diverse, our aftercare plans must again be individualized. Physicians and clinics address ongoing physical recovery based on both our specific needs and the ever evolving field of cancer care. Whether you are entering later stages of the physical journey or preparing yourself for the future, this philosophy applies equally well to our continuing social, emotional and spiritual needs.

Aftercare: Once Again, It's Physical and More

For me, the completion of primary treatment was an abrupt and somewhat confusing experience. Certainly, I was relieved to be finished with radiation and chemotherapy. I was thrilled to be given a diagnosis of full remission. Yet, it was weeks before I felt much better physically, plus the immediate disconnect from most of the medical staff that had been so pivotal in my treatment was a significant loss. I didn't miss the pain, but I most assuredly missed those angels of mercy who had been so skilled and so compassionate. I have since learned that this is not an uncommon response from survivors as we complete an intense course of treatment.

I am now several years into the aftercare process. My physical plan involves scheduled follow-up with my surgeon and radiation oncologist, along with periodic scans. Gradually I have been able to return to a normal work schedule and full participation in family life, although my pace has certainly slowed. Surgery and radiation caused changes in my physical appearance that seem more noticeable and more important to me than to those I am close to. I am reminded daily that I was treated for cancer by the scar across my neck, the tingling nerves in my shoulder and ear, my dry mouth, the serious increase in wrinkles on my face and the little tattooed dots on my chest and neck.

As mentioned, my massage therapist has helped me with the muscle hardness and discomfort I experienced due to radiation (I wish my biceps were as tight as my neck). My singing voice is slowly returning as my voice box seems to be more mobile, to use a nonclinical term. Over many months, the effects of my treatment have diminished. Unlike other survivors I know, I do not currently labor with any major limitations in physical functioning. But, I am not the same physical being post-cancer.

Many of us will need consultation on concerns about appearance, sexuality, mobility and a myriad of other aspects of ongoing physical recovery. We may need to learn how to take better care of the physical self that remains. These essential aftercare strategies can, once again, be organized with the input of knowledgeable cancer specialists.

Emotionally, I am also not the same man post-cancer. In some ways, I have evolved. I am more grateful for my life. I am more grateful for my friends and family. As I regain strength and focus, I am acutely aware of the toll my cancer took on my family, the fatigue and fear and hours of caring for me. I am less fearful of my mortality, more accepting of those I love, less judgmental of those who annoy me and less driven toward achievement. Even as someone who has always been somewhat of a 'nontraditional' man when it came to expressing emotion, I find myself even more likely to cry when happy, sad or scared.

I also find myself more anxious about the health and safety of the people I love most. At times I am more uncomfortable with conflict. Like other survivors I have spoken with, no amount of reassurance that I am currently healthy removes those moments of anxiety each time I feel a small ache or wait for the results of my latest test. Although I no longer replay the effects of treatment in my daily memory, my heart can still be moved to emotion when discussing the rigors of recovery.

Spiritually, I am more deeply convinced that life contains mysteries, challenges and miracles beyond our complete understanding. My long-held belief in the power of loving relationships has been put to the test and come up a winner. Victor Frankl, one of my psychotherapy heroes, taught that great meaning, powerful new learning and amazing acts of kindness can flow from times of pain and challenge. Cancer took me to each of these places, over and over.

And, in spite of what I have re-learned about the value of relationships in my life, on occasion I still find myself stepping away from communication and connection. A recent lunch with my old friend Doug reminded me that I had become inconsistent in making contact with some of the people I am closest to. Post-treatment, as I had returned to a more normal schedule, I had become a bit haphazard in reaching out. Having relied so heavily on my family and friends during treatment, I had apparently decided they might need a break from Chris. As I shared this awareness with Doug, I was challenged to practice what I teach: maintain contact and sustain the relationships that are not only valued by me, but by my friends.

This is my aftercare story as of today. I hope that additional insights into the impact of survivorship will trickle into my consciousness over time.

Your story of ongoing care might be quite different from mine. Perhaps you will be involved in extended care. I recently read an amazing story, written by an incredible survivor, who has been receiving cancer care for more than six years; and her treatment continues. You may be a survivor who has received more than one course of treatment, for the same or a new cancer diagnosis.

You may also have vastly different after-effects from your therapy. I have heard many stories of life changing treatment responses much more severe than my own.

What is the narrative of your ongoing recovery? What are your ongoing physical, social, emotional and spiritual needs as you move forward? Would you benefit from services to help you cope with changes in mobility, changes in physical appearance, sexual functioning, ongoing support for recovery from addictions?

Who are the people who will continue to listen to you as you make the adjustments of recovery? How will you maintain the partnerships in healing that you have worked so hard to establish during diagnosis and primary treatment?

Take the time to reflect on these questions. Take the time to evaluate the issues of nutrition, exercise, sexuality, career, finances and relationships as you move into extended care.

Your Self-Care Plan

There is an abundance of literature for survivors on managing the long-term effects of cancer and maintaining a healthy lifestyle. Books, magazine, websites and blogs offer credible strategies for nutrition, physical activity, stress management, family health and more.

For some of us, aftercare can be a return to many of the positive, health giving activities of the past. For others, recovery is an opportunity to build a new, healthier approach to daily life. Your plan may include significant restrictions that were not present in your life before a diagnosis of cancer.

Talk to your team. Discuss issues of diet, exercise, emotional health and spiritual practice. Design a personal self-care plan that meets your unique ongoing needs. If you are so inclined, write it down.

And, as always, remember that we are works in progress. The plan can continue to evolve. Last year, I wrote a book. This year, I'm back on my bicycle, dry mouth and all. Who knows what next year might bring.

Time Does Not March On

A common thread that runs through the conversations of many people who have suffered a loss or major change is the sense that "Other people have moved on; I guess I need to." This does not necessarily mean that folks have truly moved forward in their hearts and minds. This is a message about deciding "Not to bother people." In a self-critical view, lingering in the emotion sparked by past events can be seen as (ma)lingering, rather than a normal and necessary stage in healing.

Statements I have heard on numerous occasions, uttered by folks who are continuing to cope with a life altering experience, include:

"I need to just get over it."

"Other people have it a lot worse than me. I need to move on."

"I need to quit whining."

"People are probably tired of hearing from me."

"I need to suck it up."

"Life goes on."

I'd like to offer an alternative view, one that both honors the importance of moving forward and recognizes that the journey through cancer is not attached to any specific timeline:

Indeed, life does go on. However, this does not mean that the effects of certain life occurrences can simply be turned off with the flick of a switch.

Cancer is not an event. Cancer is a process, a series of moments crowded with ambiguity, intense emotion, setbacks and celebrations that demand an extended period of contemplation and communication with trusted advocates.

Some of us do not simply enter aftercare, per se. Your experience may be that of long-term, periodic or constant care. It is essential to stay open to support as you move forward.

A strong social system also recognizes a family's continued need for social, emotional and spiritual support, as survivors integrate the changes brought forth by cancer.

As with earlier stages of recovery, it is possible to be independent and strong while simultaneously creating space for others to advise and assist us in the aftercare phase. At some point, cancer may not command the same level of attention in your internal life that it did during diagnosis, primary treatment and early recovery. Yet even at this stage, recovery is steady movement, not a sprint to some imaginary finish line.

Take time to weave your path through cancer into the larger fabric of your life. Once again, we are not defined by this illness, nor does healing mean that your cancer experience disappears as if it never existed.

Caregivers Also Need Time to Recover

Each member of the survivor's team has walked a physically, emotionally and spiritually exhausting road. Perhaps you, as an advocate, have made time for your own health and healing during treatment and early recovery. Perhaps you have focused primarily on the needs of the survivor and on the responsibilities thrust upon you by his or her cancer. Many of you remain in a caregiver role.

In any event, you too require time to replenish your resources and reconcile the ways in which cancer has impacted your life. Consider these questions:

> Are there feelings or concerns that you have withheld from your survivor during the most crucial stages of treatment, protecting him or her from the stress? Would it be helpful for you to discuss any of these issues as you venture together into the aftercare phase?

> Are there activities that create intimacy and connection with your loved ones that were, necessarily, set aside at earlier stages of treatment? What old pleasures would you like to return to? What new adventures would you like to pursue?

> As treatment continues for the survivor in your life, is there unfinished business: practical, emotional or spiritual issues that demand your time and energy? Are there plans to be made that will provide you and your family with a greater degree of security as medical intervention continues?

> Do you need time alone to rest, relax, meditate and recreate? When will you take that time?

> Do you need time with important people in your support system to reconnect, rejuvenate, celebrate and grieve? Who are these people? When will you take that time?

Answering these questions is not intended to create within you a sense of obligation, or a new to-do list. More chores you do not need. Rather, taking time to identify the activities and people who help you refill your tank, or bring you a greater degree of security and peace.

Time to Grieve

Since ending primary treatment I have attended services for three survivors who have passed. Each of these incredible individuals had caring people who followed them to the last step in their journey through cancer.

I have friends who have initiated their first treatment and several who have re-entered treatment. These courageous survivors inspire me with an amazing combination of independent will, faith and a reliance on the best of caregivers.

Sorrow and setbacks are common companions with hope and gratitude as we continue down the path of recovery. Healing does not always mean cured. At times, it means grieving the loss of someone dear to us after weeks, months or even years of care giving and advocacy. It may mean grieving the loss of functioning that cancer and cancer treatment can bring.

I do not offer a specific method for grief resolution within these pages. There are numerous resources to help those of us who face the loss of a loved one. But, I will offer a simple formula for grief that I have used for years:

The Size of My Grief = The Size of My Love

Grief reminds us of the value of people in our lives when we experience loss. This is not wrong, it is normal. And much like other aspects of cancer care, healing for this grief is available to each of us.

I have often said to clients in need of consolation that grief is universal. Although many people have not lost a loved one to cancer, the world is full of compassionate individuals who have experienced some substantial loss in their lives. They understand the shock, sadness, anger and confusion that often accompany death and dying. They understand that grief involves weeks, months, even years of emotion and adjustment. Some of these people are professionals, specialists in grief therapy. As previously discussed, some will be those natural healers, good listeners who bring an open heart to our struggle. For many of us, new friends, people who understand the cancer journey, will assist us in times of loss and grief.

I believe that grief often also contains some aspect of celebration, the recognition of a life well spent. We celebrate with tears and stories. We pay tribute to survivors with memories of their lives and the hope of our own healing. We honor the community of caring by sharing our pain with those who understand.

Time to Celebrate

Celebrating life can also take many forms. Whoop and holler. Dance. Skydive. Write a book.

Celebrating recovery from cancer is, at least in part, a community process. It's vital that we make merry with our spouses and life partners, immediate family, small and large gatherings of extended family and friends, and often, with other folks whose lives have been affected by cancer.

I vividly remember attending my first survivors' event. I told my story. I heard the stories of other survivors and caregivers. Some of the memories were overflowing with joy, some were very sad. All were celebrations of the lives of courageous people. We laughed, we commiserated, we hugged, some of us cried. I found three new friends that day, not knowing we would soon join one another in volunteer work.

Throughout these pages, I have invited you to allow people to support you in the most difficult days of recovery even if you are, by nature, a private or solitary person. Let the same be true when you experience any measure of loss, or victory over cancer. Certainly, feel the joy in the quiet of your own thoughts and heart. Share a silent prayer of thanks with your Higher Power. And then, break out the nutritious snacks and connect with your loved ones!

Gratitude: An Opportunity to Give Back

As previously mentioned, a second theme that flows through the narratives of many survivors and family members I have met is the profound sense of appreciation felt toward the caregivers who have been the most sensitive and responsive during the ordeal of treatment. Certainly, folks are extremely grateful for the knowledge and skill of medical staff and the technical assistance of other talented advocates. Yet the stories I hear often focus most intensely on those people who listened, answered important questions, smiled, communicated respectfully, expressed genuine empathy and took decisive action.

Expressing our Gratitude

If you are one of those grateful survivors and advocates, I encourage you to translate appreciation into action.

Here are a few ideas:

Write a thank-you letter to the director of your clinic or the CEO of the hospital where you received exceptional service. Be specific. Let them know what you found most helpful. Name names; let them know which staff provided the best care.

Write a thank-you letter to the staff members who cared for you. Again, tell them what part of their service was most valuable to you and your loved ones.

Write a "Letter to the Editor" of your local newspaper. Whether or not it gets published, send a copy to your clinic and hospital.

Bring a small token of appreciation to the staff when you go for follow-up care: a card, food, a bouquet, or maybe just a big smile.

Make a donation to cancer care or another charity in the name of particular staff, your clinic, or hospital. Make sure they are notified that a contribution was made in honor of their hard work.

Attend an event for cancer survivors and family. Tell the people you meet about the wonderful caregivers you have met in your journey.

What are your ideas about creatively expressing your appreciation to the professionals who best exemplify a high level of compassionate and skilled care?

Volunteerism: Another Form of Gratitude

There is no more active way to express our thanks than to offer our time and energy to a cause that holds meaning in our lives. The volunteerism I have observed in cancer care is nothing short of amazing.

Nearly two dozen survivors, family members and professionals volunteered to join the initial Patient and Family Advisory Council organized by my clinic. As I write, I am sipping water from the really cool mug embossed with our really cool logo. I am aware, just within my immediate circle, of folks who are coordinating cancer fund raisers, providing support to breast and prostate cancer survivors, participating in cancer prevention events, promoting support groups for child and adult survivors, and simply being available for emotional and spiritual support to survivors and advocates as they move through the various stages of cancer.

Opportunities are boundless for participation in the mission of curing cancer and easing the suffering of all those affected by this illness. And that is just cancer care.

There is no rule that our gratitude must be expressed through service that is specific to healing cancer. Perhaps you are already actively involved in other volunteer efforts and will bring an even deeper passion to your work.

If you are uncertain about the direction your service might take, I encourage you to take a few minutes to answer these questions:

What issues are you most passionate about in your life (cancer care, poverty, healthcare, child abuse prevention, addictions, education)?

What people are you most passionate about in your life (children, families, the elderly, the mentally ill, the addicted, the physically ill)?

What skills and talents do you have that would assist others in volunteer settings (remember, time and energy alone are of great value)?

In what capacity would you be willing and able to serve as a volunteer?

If you are uncertain about the specific needs in your community, I suggest one or more of the following:

Contact your local United Way and learn about the myriad of nonprofit groups that need volunteers in your community.

Contact a church of your choosing for information about programs offered by the religious community for those in need.

Connect with the Volunteer Coordinator of your local hospital or clinic.

If you are involved in Alcoholics Anonymous or another 12 Step recovery program, reach out to a local addictions treatment center or correctional facility and offer yourself in service.

For some of us the ongoing challenges of cancer, the aftercare process or other physical concerns may limit our ability to volunteer. I want each of you to know that you will be presented with opportunities to serve, if even for a brief moment.

Three days after leaving ICU, I was slowly motoring down the hallway. I met a man shuffling the other direction. He was a fellow throat cancer survivor. We spoke briefly and offered mutual words of encouragement. Neither of us was feeling very well, but it was a powerful moment of mutual support.

Whatever your interests or energy there are people who are hungry for your gifts. We have faced cancer. We have learned that we are not alone. Let's pass it on.

Last and Most: Appreciation of Family and Friends

As I draw the first draft this book to a close I am sitting in an exquisite retreat center, the Cave House. This facility was the vision of Jim Armour, a man I never met. I am sitting at my computer in the Sunrise Room, overlooking the Ohio River on an unusually warm and breezy day in February. His dream, alive long after his transition, allows folks like me to create in wondrous solitude.

And in this quiet, as the barges silently drift down river, what are my most powerful thoughts? My mind turns to family and friends. They are with me, even as I sit alone.

DiAnne will be at work, passionately dedicating another day to the lives of disadvantaged children, soon to return home as the coolest mom I have ever known. She is one of my heroes. Nathan, an amazing young man and a wise soul, is discovering the wonders of classic literature, music and his own devotion to a spiritual life. Aimee, my role model of the open heart, will be planning the heck out of another community event in the beautiful town where she lives, then, maybe meeting one or more of her friends for dinner and a movie. Will Carly, who embodies the value of friendship, be heading to work, working out, socializing, or all of the above today?

My friends and other family members will be teaching school, leading men's groups, counseling, working for hospice, attending to brand new grandbabies, playing with their children, tending to sick loved ones, or just soaking up the balmy day.

Those I love most will be in relationship, continuing to give and take the greatest gift we have as human beings. Connection.

In community, we can live our lives to the fullest. We can bring hope to others in need. We can be the caregivers and advocates for others when their times of challenge come.

We can go forward with open hearts.

ABOUT THE AUTHOR

Chris Frey, MSW, ACSW, LCSW; psychotherapist, author, teacher, and Stage 4 throat and neck cancer survivor is in private practice in St. Louis, MO. For several decades, Chris has been a leading voice in men's issues, addiction recovery, relationships and sexuality. His work in sexual addiction, expressive therapy, healthy masculinity and, most recently, collaborative cancer care has kept him on the front lines of innovation in emotional healing work.

As a cancer survivor and author, Chris was the recipient of an Armour Foundation sabbatical, in 2009, which assists in funding creative works. From this sabbatical sprung, *I'm Sorry, It's Cancer: A Handbook of Help and Hope for Survivors and Caregivers.* An excerpt of his book is featured in the January-February 2010 issue of *Coping with Cancer* magazine.

Chris' advocacy for survivors has included serving as the co-chair of the Patient and Family Advisory Council of the Siteman Cancer Center: Barnes-St. Peters. Chris and his wife, DiAnne, were recorded as part of the StoryCorps Archive series. Their interview on the effects of a cancer diagnosis is entered, alongside other families, in the American Folklife Center at the Library of Congress. His presentations on supportive cancer care have included Southeastern Illinois College and the Barnes-St. Peters Cancer Survivors Day.

Chris is the author of two critically praised books, *Men at Work: An Action Guide to Masculine Healing* and *Double Jeopardy: Treating Male Juvenile Sex Offenders/Substance Abusers*, and the co-author of *FatherTime: Stories on the Heart and Soul of Fathering* with Chris Scribner, PhD. His articles have been published in both professional and popular journals, including *Social Work, GP Solo, the Missouri Bar Journal* and *Everyman.*

For many years Chris has been a popular workshop leader and nationally recognized speaker on topics as diverse as masculinity, sexual and chemical addictions, healthy sexuality and healthy relationships. He is a past presenter at the Chicago Men's Conference, the National Conference on Sexual Addiction and Compulsivity, the

Heartland Men's Conference and the Missouri Lawyer's Assistance Conference. Chris is a member of the Academy of Certified Social Workers and the Society for the Advancement of Sexual Health.

Most important, Chris is a husband and the father of three young adults. In his spare time he is both a passionate and mediocre guitarist.

CONTACT INFORMATION

Additional copies of *I'm Sorry, It's Cancer* can be purchased at www.Lulu.com or www.amazon.com.

I can be reached for workshop and presentation requests at:

Chris Frey, MSW, LCSW
Frey and Tobin Counseling Associates
933 Gardenview Office Parkway
St. Louis, MO 63141
(314) 997-1403

or through my website at:
www.chrisfreycounseling.com